# Rule a Healthy Roost

*Nutrition, Recipes, and Activities for Modern Families*

## by Leslie Smith Grant

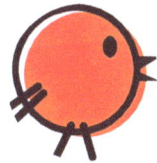

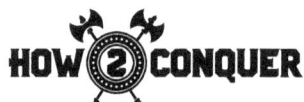

**HOW 2 CONQUER**

Published by How2Conquer
1990 Hosea L. Williams Drive NE
Atlanta, Georgia 30317
www.how2conquer.com

First edition, 2008
Second edition, 2020

Cover illustrations by Kelly Giardino
Interior design by Emily Owens
Edited by Katherine Guntner

Illustrations by Natalya Levish

Table of Contents photo by Seedjan
Page 1 photo by Candace Bond
Page 2 photo by Lelia Milaya
Page 8 photo by Katie Mayne
Page 10 photo by Felix Cesare
Page 15 photo by Michelle Patrick
Page 17 photo by Tiffany Egbert
Pages 39 and 61 photos by Natasa Goras
Pages 47 and 79 photos by Nata Bene
Page 50 photo by Christina Kooiker
Page 74 photo by Nicole Nelson
Page 88 photo by Maryna Voronova
Page 91 photo by Tasha Kandaurova
Page 97 photo by Crystal Sing
Page 110 photo by Olga Polishko
Page 125 photo by Carina König
Page 129 photo by Petch
Page 139 photo by Talent Zukutu
Page 145 photo by Mikey Lane

Printed in the United States of America

Library of Congress Control Number: 2020935887

Print ISBN 978-1-945783-05-0
Ebook ISBN 978-1-945783-06-7

This book is dedicated to
all the little "chickins" with love and
hope for a most healthy future!

And to Anne J. Smith

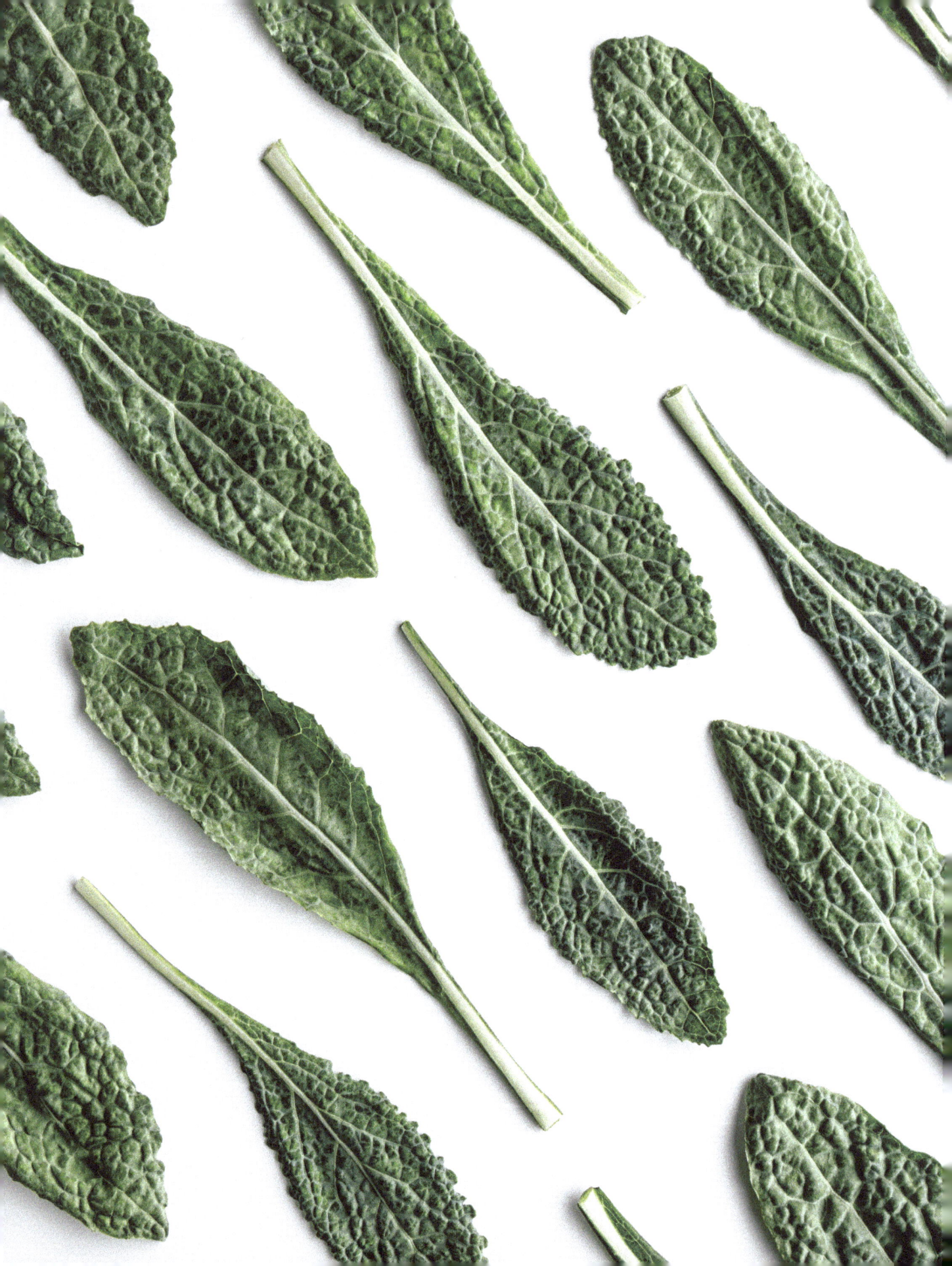

# Table of Contents

# Introduction

*Rule a Healthy Roost* is based on a collection of works by myself and an incredibly creative bunch called The Chickin Coop (bios in the About Us section), which was initially published in 2008 under the name *The Chickin Feed Primer*. We thought How2Conquer was a great fit to scatter these ideas in 2020!

The idea for this book started when I became very frustrated with the daily struggle of what to feed my kids. My lack of nutrition knowledge was deeply rooted. Our family joke growing up was that we knew what was for dinner when we could see the color of the bag (we ate a lot of fast food!). Not wanting to pass along this "food apathy" to my children, I set about searching for a simple and fun way to access good nutrition information.

This guide gives an essential understanding of what a balanced diet looks like, what portion sizes should be, and why each of the food groups we eat are important. It's a simple, fun book that is meant to be shared with your kids. We hope it will serve as an introduction (or revisit if needed) to a healthy lifestyle. It covers just the basics – nothing too difficult to understand – for creating a healthy kitchen and home. We've also provided some fun ways to keep your kids active and great resources to further the mission.

We've worked to cover just enough to get you interested in some very important subjects, which you can delve into more deeply as needed. *Rule a Healthy Roost* is consciously designed to evoke a simpler time, back when decisions about what to eat were simpler. You ate what was fresh and available – fast food and the mass-marketing of sugared-up "foods" had not yet occurred, and the idea of an obesity epidemic was unthinkable. Kids ran around all day, did their chores, and played outside until dark. They weren't in front of a TV or computer screen all day.

A group of very talented moms and a P.E. Coach assembled this book to be a simple reference that can be shared with all members of the family. It's not meant to be an academic tome on nutrition, a complete recipe book, or a fitness text. It will provide some starting points for each of these areas. We hope that you will supplement the information in this book by investigating the websites and books listed in the reference section – once you get the basics down.

From the early stages it was clear that I was not alone in my desire to give my kids a nutritional "leg-up." We have heard from families all around the globe that are desperate to re-educate their children. After sharing the prototype of the Nutrition Tracking Board with a nutritionist who said, "I've never seen anything like this – what a great idea," we began looking in earnest at how to explain the concepts behind these tracking boards.

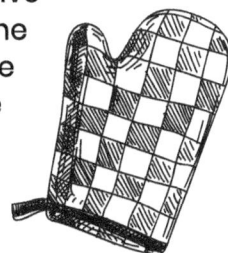

We knew it would be helpful to put together information that gives a better (and more thorough) explanation of the different foods we should eat each day and why they are important. With this in mind, our goals were to:

1.  Include some yummy recipes to demonstrate how foods are put together and how the food on our plates relates to recommended daily portions.

2.  Throw in some good "mom-sense" to keep in mind while you are shopping and planning your kitchen.

3.  Provide some fun ways to keep our kids active.

We're on a mission to help busy modern families keep nutrition and fitness a priority in their daily lives. We hope *Rule a Healthy Roost* will become a helpful tool in teaching your kids the importance of good nutrition and their own role in making healthy choices.

## Tracking Goals: Simple, fun, effective solutions

Before making the Nutrition Tracking Board, I'd never seen anything like it. I knew about the Food Pyramid. It was taped onto the back of the cafeteria door at Idlewood Elementary School in Tucker, GA. Obviously it made some kind of impression since I recall it 30 years later. It seemed like straight forward enough advice. So when I went looking for a good teaching tool for myself and my kids, the Food Pyramid came to mind.

It suggested how much of each food category you should have each day to get a balanced diet. That seemed simple, but it was terribly un-fun, and you had to keep up with what you had eaten all day long – too much for my "mom brain."

I know that keeping a "food journal" has been successful for many folks who can stay on a diet. The concept of tracking food is not new, and there are many ways to do it. I found lots of other great information about nutrition, but little that was interactive – save for apps and online options. I really didn't want to increase the amount of time we spent in front of a screen!

In order for it to work for our family, it had to be something we could see without having to log on or find said "food journal" (that the dog inevitably chewed up yesterday) and a pencil (ditto about the dog).

For our new "nutrition training" to be effective, I needed to come up with some way to put the basic information in a practical format that could be readily accessed. It also had to be something that was nice to look at so we would pay attention to it, and if it was well-designed we wouldn't mind giving up some of the visual real estate in our kitchen. (Not that I'm that picky, but the front of our fridge already looks like the junk drawer threw up on it.) So I set about to find an "in-your-face format" that was designed to be in the kitchen, 24/7.

# HOW 2 CONQUER

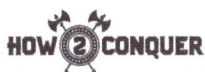

# Rule a Healthy Roost

## Nutrition Tracking

| They Need | | Nutrition Tracking | They've Had | |
|---|---|---|---|---|
| **Grains/Bread/Pasta** | | Serving: 1 slice bread; ½ cup cooked rice, pasta, or cereal — Total: 5 oz daily | **Grains/Bread/Pasta** | |
| **Veggies** | | Serving: ½ cup each — Total: 1½–2 cups daily | **Veggies** | |
| **Fruits** | | Serving: ½ cup each — Total: 1½ cups daily | **Fruits** | |
| **Dairy** | | Serving: ⅔ cup each — Total: 2 cups daily | **Dairy** | |
| **Protein (Fish/Meat/Beans)** | | Serving: 1 oz meat, 1 egg, 1 Tbsp peanut butter, or ¼ cup dry beans — Total: 4–5 oz equivalents daily | **Protein (Fish/Meat/Beans)** | |
| **Activity (Running, Jumping, Playing)** | | Get out and PLAY! | **Activity (Running, Jumping, Playing)** | |
| **Sweets & Extras** | | Our bodies don't need these, but sometimes our minds do. If it doesn't fit above, it goes here. | **Sweets & Extras** | |

**This board belongs to:**

*Amounts shown are based upon recommendations by the USDA for 3–8 year olds. For variations and more specific info, visit www.mypyramid.gov.

The Rule a Healthy Roost Nutrition Tracking Board is available for download from the How2Conquer website. It's designed for children ages 3–8, but kids of any age can use the board – just go to www.choosemyplate.gov/MyPlatePlan and plug in your info if it differs from the Tracking Board. Remember, kids and their parents can have a range of nutrient needs depending on their age, physical activity level, and gender.

The first step was to break down the balanced diet into its component parts (serving-sized portions for each food category). The second step was to arrange them in a simple way so we could see what we needed and what we'd actually had each day, like a chore chart. This would allow us to mark off or track when something had been eaten, and I could keep up with our progress and plan better meals.

I started out with a rudimentary board and soon had a "Eureka!" moment. This board would not only help me keep up with what I was serving, but more importantly, it would also be a simple way for my kids to keep up with what they were eating. They could easily learn about what their daily eating should look like, what they really needed versus what they wanted, and they would be able to keep track of it themselves.

## Visual Guide

The Rule a Healthy Roost Nutrition Tracking Board was invented to help families learn together about healthy eating. The Tracking Board provides both active and passive learning for your family. The kids can actively be involved in making choices and moving their markers, and the board continually serves as a passive reminder of their goals.

The Tracking Board provides two identical columns: the left side is what they need each day, and the right side is what they've actually had. Children are involved in tracking their food choices by figuring out what they are eating (parents, this is a wonderful learning opportunity to talk about your mouthfuls!) and then marking them on the board.

One of the nicest side effects of the board is that it takes the pressure off parents to have to conjure up endless explanations about why kids have to eat their veggies! Just have them check out their boards and see what they've had for the day. "See that lonely little veggie oven mitt? He wants to join his friends – please help him." Who says a little bit o' guilt isn't a wonderful thing sometimes?

When using your Tracking Board to log your progress, know that it is designed to help you get the recommended variety of foods without making things too difficult or confusing. If you aren't certain which category the foods you are eating fit into, be flexible! Consider what you need overall for the day and move two markers for something if need be. For example, many dairy products are high in protein, so you could move two magnets (Dairy and Protein) for the one serving. If your dairy product is a milkshake, then be sure to move your Sweets & Extras magnet too, since milkshakes are high in fat and sugar. A milkshake has calcium and protein, but it also has much more fat and sugar than a cup of 1% milk.

I hope you will find this updated version helpful for you and your family.

– Leslie Smith Grant

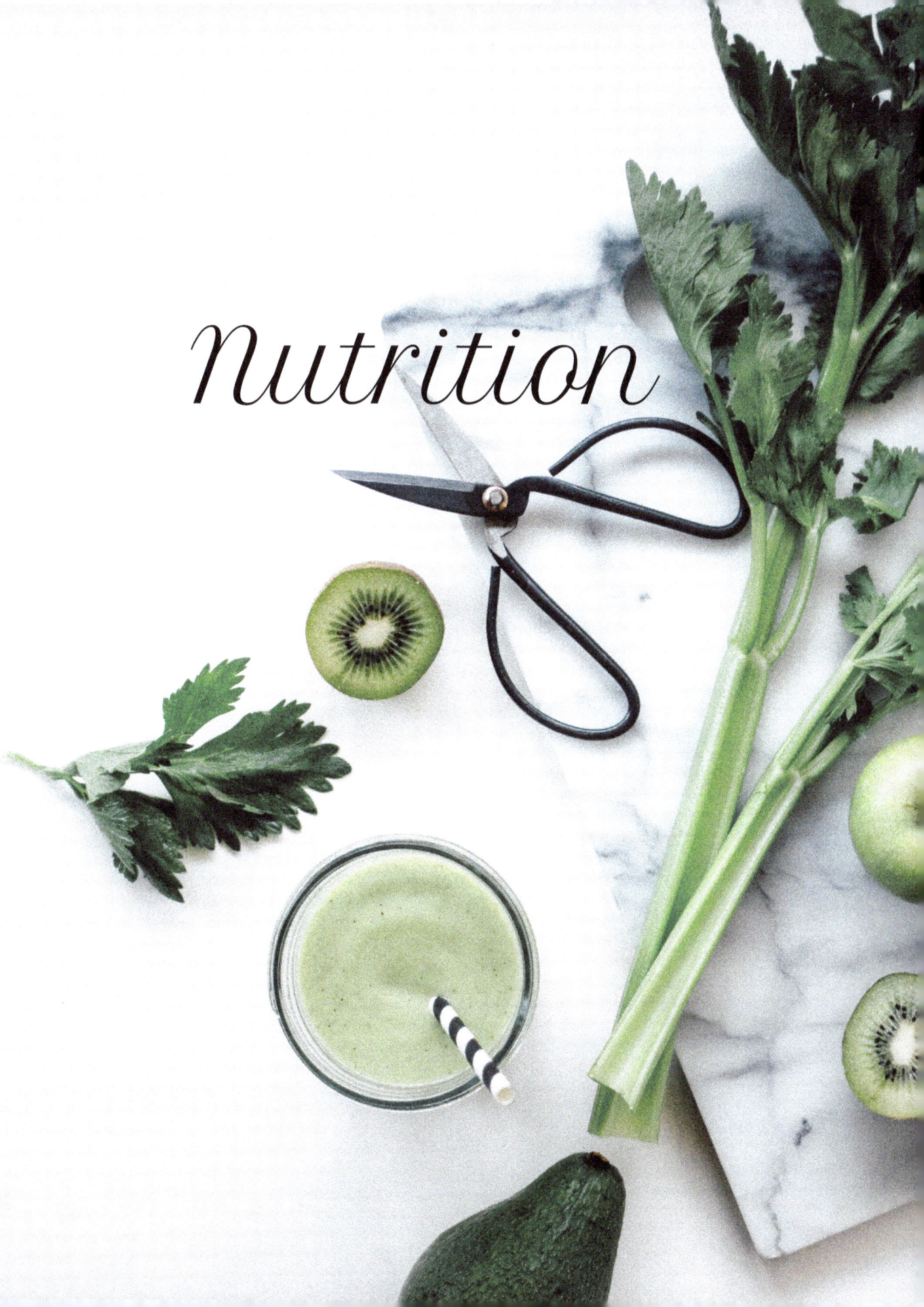

# Nutrition

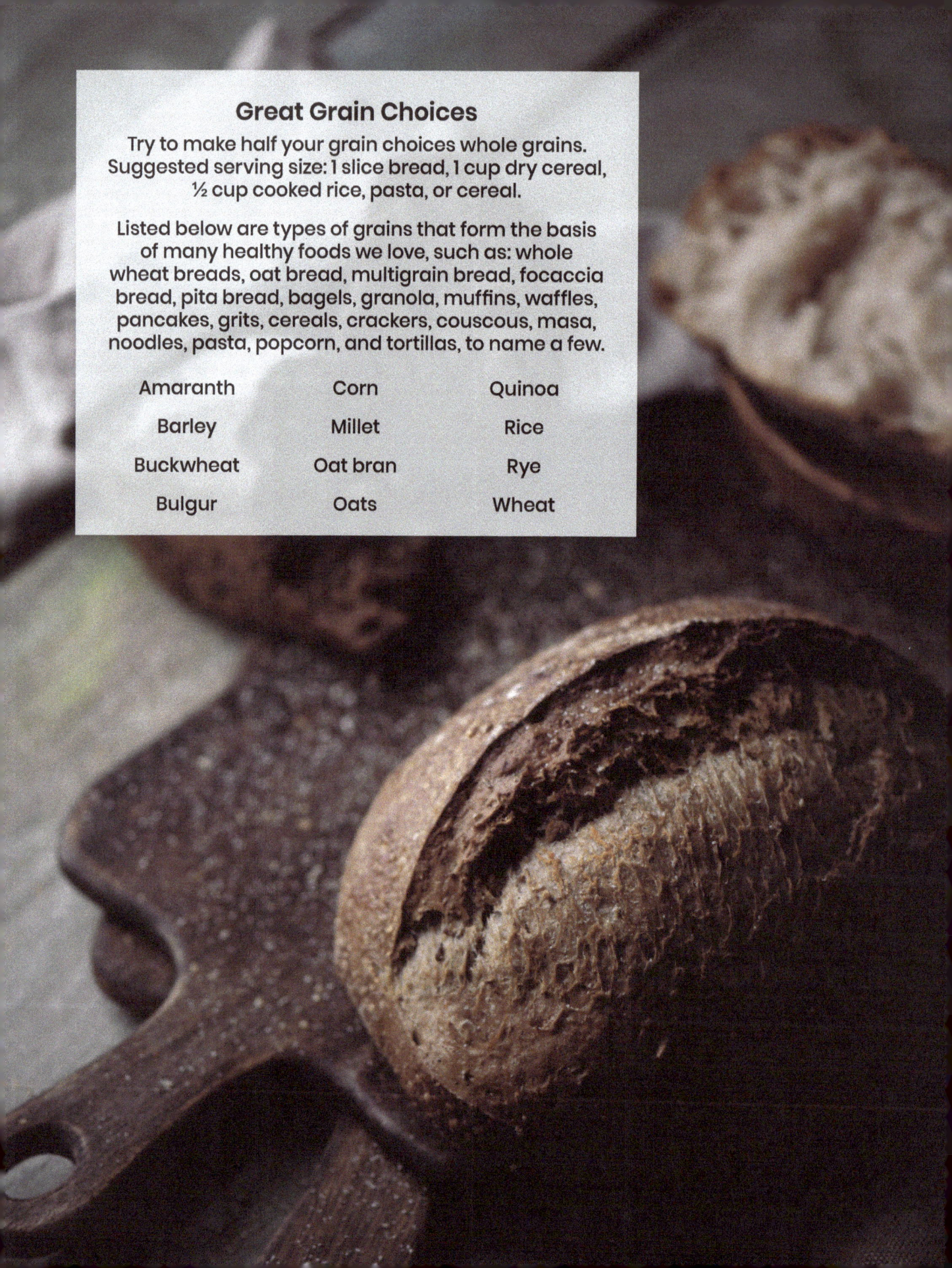

## Great Grain Choices

Try to make half your grain choices whole grains. Suggested serving size: 1 slice bread, 1 cup dry cereal, ½ cup cooked rice, pasta, or cereal.

Listed below are types of grains that form the basis of many healthy foods we love, such as: whole wheat breads, oat bread, multigrain bread, focaccia bread, pita bread, bagels, granola, muffins, waffles, pancakes, grits, cereals, crackers, couscous, masa, noodles, pasta, popcorn, and tortillas, to name a few.

| | | |
|---|---|---|
| Amaranth | Corn | Quinoa |
| Barley | Millet | Rice |
| Buckwheat | Oat bran | Rye |
| Bulgur | Oats | Wheat |

# Grains/Bread/Pasta

## Yum… good old comforting carbohydrates.

This category has received a bad rap in recent years, but kids (and adults) need this vital source of readily available energy.

Whole grains are sources of fiber, vitamins, and complex carbohydrates, which are important for good health and sustained energy. Kids ages four to eight (4–8) should be getting about 25 grams of fiber a day from grains, beans/legumes, fruits, and vegetables (check food labels and use your Nutrition Tracking Board to keep up). Key nutrients also found in grains are iron and the B vitamins niacin, thiamin, and riboflavin. Many store-bought breads are now fortified with folate.

Nutrition experts recommend that half of your grain sources be whole grain. The grains group can be very healthy depending on how they are prepared. For example, enjoy pasta with a little olive oil or tomato sauce instead of a cream sauce. Sandwiches can be just as yummy on whole grain bread without the extra mayonnaise – you can try out different mustards or some yummy hummus (see the recipe section). Fiber is listed on food labels, so check before you buy.

## Some suggestions:

Buy whole grains. Breads, flours, cereals, pastas, rice, and tortillas all come in whole grain varieties. Mix them ½ and ½ to start with if you need to ease into it.

## Flours and Breads

- Check your grocery store for whole grain and whole wheat options, like bread, tortillas, pizza crusts, and waffles.

- Many commercially made breads have slices that are larger than recommended portion sizes. Use a large cookie cutter to cut fun shapes and make kid-sized sandwiches.

- On a day when you have more time, make waffles or pancakes with whole wheat flour. You can also get creative and make oat cakes or muffins. Kids love them, and they can be frozen for a quick healthy breakfast on busy mornings.

- Even pizza, the tried-and-true kid favorite, can be made with whole wheat crust.

- Buckwheat noodles, also called soba noodles, make a yummy base for an asian-flavored veggie stir fry, steamed vegetables, or soup.

## Grains

- Enjoy hearty brown rice instead of white rice. Make plenty and keep it in the fridge to serve over a few days.

- Eat cereals that say whole grain. If your kids balk at the high fiber cereal, try mixing a whole grain, high fiber cereal with their favorite.

- Make a steaming bowl of oatmeal and add fruit. (But watch for instant oatmeal in packets – lots of added sugar!)

- Some granola bars are made with whole grains (check the ingredient list). These can be less healthy than their reputation suggests due to high sugar. For example, some granola bars may be labeled "natural" but still include as much as seven forms of sugar! Yikes! High fructose corn syrup or high maltose corn syrup are other types of sweeteners. Best to avoid these as much as possible.

- Quinoa is a grain that has a wonderful texture, absorbs flavors beautifully, and is a complete protein. It's the most ancient of all grains and has been cultivated for 5,000 years. Quinoa is called the "mother grain" from Chile to the Peruvian Andes.

- Couscous is teeny tiny pasta that cooks in 5 minutes. Throw some veggies in while it is cooking, and voila! You have part of your healthy dinner done fast and with only one pot to wash.

- Barley is a source of fiber and iron, and it's a delicious addition to soups or salads.

- Alternatives for gluten intolerant folks include flours made from corn, quinoa, rice, potatoes, and soy.

## What about gluten free?

Gluten is a term that describes tiny parts (specific amino acid sequences) of a group of proteins. Gluten can be found in products containing wheat, rye, and barley. Avoiding gluten means no breads, cereals, pastas, baked goods, or any food product with wheat on the food label. This also means no wheat starch, wheat germ, bran, triticale, bulgur, spelt, and malt flavoring.

Substitutions include potato products, corn, rice, soybeans, amaranth, millet, tapioca, and arrowroot. A small amount of oats may be tolerated by some gluten-free eaters.

## Why would someone need to avoid gluten?

A gluten-free diet is the best known treatment for celiac disease, an autoimmune condition in which the body reacts to gluten like it's a foreign invader. Damage to the intestines results, causing pain, bloating, and a reduced ability to absorb some nutrients. Symptoms improve when a strict gluten-free diet is followed.

Since products with gluten are such staples of a typical American diet, a registered dietitian should be consulted if you or your a child has celiac disease.

You may have heard that a gluten-free and/or a casein-free diet is helpful for kids with autistic spectrum disorder. Much of the information out there is anecdotal (not proven or entirely reliable). Currently there are few high quality, blinded, placebo-controlled studies that can clearly demonstrate whether or not this diet is beneficial to kids with autism. We just don't know yet if this restrictive type of diet can give families the answers they are seeking. More studies are surely needed.

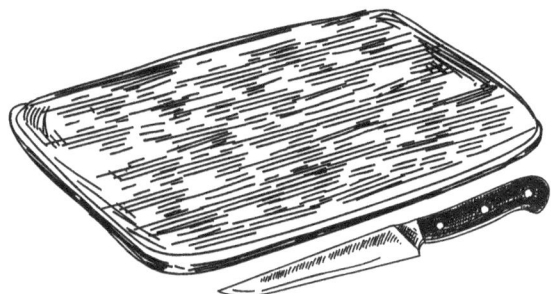

# Veggies

**I imagine you've heard over and over that we need to eat our veggies.**

Why are they so important? Veggies are a great source of many vitamins, including vitamins A and C, which are important for good vision, growth, healing, tissue repair, bone, and tooth health – not to mention these vitamins improve resistance to infections.

Veggies, especially colorful ones, contain antioxidants that may help in the prevention of some chronic diseases such as cancer and heart disease. Kids who are introduced to veggies early on are much more likely to have healthy eating habits as adolescents and adults. Veggies are naturally low in fat, cholesterol, and sugar. They add color, texture, and taste to dishes.

Great news for busy families: fresh is best, but frozen is fine. Don't worry if you don't have time to prepare only fresh veggies. Going for frozen can be just as healthy.

Go easy on the canned veggies though, as they can be high in salt and the nutrient content may be affected. Choose a variety of colorful veggies each week, and don't be afraid to experiment. Busy kids have a hard enough time getting one serving of veggies in, so how can you help them get the recommended 1 ½–2 cups daily?

## *Some suggestions:*

- Add broccoli, red pepper, or another favorite veggie to pizza.

- Cook carrots, zucchini, mushrooms, peppers, onions, etc., into your pasta sauces and make a lovely lasagna.

- Enjoy salads with dark leafy greens. Kids hate salad? Add some avocado, almonds, or walnuts. These are a tasty addition and provide healthy unsaturated fats.

- Add fresh spinach to tacos, burritos, or wraps.

### A SPECIAL NOTE ABOUT IRON:

Iron is especially important for growing children and pregnant or lactating women. While animal products provide a form of iron that the body can absorb and use easily, many plants contain iron as well.

For example, the iron in raw spinach is bound to a naturally occurring substance called oxalic acid. Gently steaming or blanching spinach helps to free the iron and make it more absorbable. The same goes for other greens. Use a variety of food preparation methods when you eat dark leafy greens to maximize the full potential of these super foods.

Other plant sources for iron include tofu, beans, and dried fruit. Including a source of vitamin C in your iron-rich meal will help with iron absorption.

- Pop some spinach leaves in a blender with your favorite smoothie ingredients. You could call these brownish/green smoothies "swamp juice."

- Top baked potatoes with a veggie stir fry. Prepare with 1–2 tablespoons of canola oil, and go easy on or eliminate sour cream.

- Be careful not to overcook veggies. Kids are sensitive to texture, and nobody likes mushy veggies. This will also minimize vitamin loss through cooking.

- Cook spinach and other greens by quickly blanching in hot water. This will make them less bitter, but it will also make the iron more absorbable. Kids are more sensitive to bitter tastes than adults.

- Take your kids to the farmers' market. Getting them involved in choosing and preparing food will encourage them to eat more veggies.

## Start a Veggie Habit

Don't worry if your kids turn their noses up at the first bite of a new veggie or fruit. You may need to introduce a new food ten to twenty times before kids decide it's not so bad (they might even like it). Once your kids are accustomed to eating dark green salads, the old iceberg lettuce just won't be as good anymore.

Demonstrate a positive attitude about fruits and veggies in front of your kids, but don't beat yourself up if your family doesn't have the perfect diet. Each day brings new opportunities to make good choices.

## Great Veggie Choices

The more colorful the better!
Suggested serving size: ½ cup (1 ½ to 2 cups daily).

| | | | | | |
|---|---|---|---|---|---|
| Artichokes | Cabbage | Ginger | Mushrooms | Potatoes | Sprouts |
| Asparagus | Carrots | Green onions | Okra | Pumpkin | Squash |
| Bamboo shoots | Cassava | Greens | Olives | Radishes | Taro |
| Basil | Celery | Jerusalem artichoke | Onions | Rhubarb | Tarragon |
| Bay leaves | Cilantro/coriander | Jicama | Oregano | Rosemary | Tomatillos |
| Beans* | Corn | Kohlrabi | Palm hearts | Rutabaga | Tomatoes |
| Beets | Cucumber | Leeks | Parsley | Sage | Turnips |
| Broccoli | Dill | Lemongrass | Parsnips | Scallions | Water chestnuts |
| Brussels sprouts | Eggplant | Mint | Peas | Seaweed | Zucchini |
| | Fennel | | Peppers | Soybeans* (edamame) | |

*Great sources of protein too!

# Fruits

## Sweet, delicious, and best of all... portable.

Fruit is the ultimate snack-on-the-go, which is good news for busy families. You can move your little tracking marker over with a serving of fresh fruit, dried fruit, fruit juice, or canned fruit.

Elementary school children should aim for 1 ½ cups a day. This category provides fiber, potassium, and vitamins such as A, C, and folate. These nutrients help keep vision sharp and teeth and gums healthy, strengthen blood vessels, repair wounds, and aid in iron absorption. Antioxidants such as beta-carotene and compounds like lycopene may help reduce the risk of cancer and help the body's immune system.

Fruit is low in calories but big on taste. Research is just beginning to reveal the power of berries and other brightly colored fruits.

While juice can be a part of a healthy diet, it is better to go easy on it due to the calories from sugar. Six to eight (6-8) ounces a day is plenty – try to add ½ cup water to ½ cup juice. (Remember you are setting their taste level and sugar expectations with what you give. The "watered down" version of juice will be perfectly acceptable if it is what they are introduced to early on).

Make sure your kids don't have the mistaken impression that they can drink an entire bottle of fruit juice "because it's good for me." They need whole fruits – and not all of that sugar! Whole fruit has fiber, which is important for a healthy gut.

## Some suggestions:

- Wash and prepare fruit ahead of time so kids have something healthy to reach for at snack time. Grapes can be kept in a bowl in the refrigerator or frozen in the freezer.

- Whole apples, oranges, bananas, and tangerines don't need refrigeration and can be easily added to lunches. Lunch studies have shown that kids are more likely to eat fruit if it is easy. For example, peeled orange slices are less likely to end up in the cafeteria trash can than a whole unpeeled orange. Once you peel them, store in a small, reusable container, and keep them cool!

- Add fruit to cereal, oatmeal, yogurt, or smoothies. Fruits headed past ripe? Put them in the freezer and use later for smoothies!

- Have fruit for dessert. Drizzle a tablespoon of chocolate syrup over a banana or strawberries for a quick, lower calorie, chocolatey dessert.

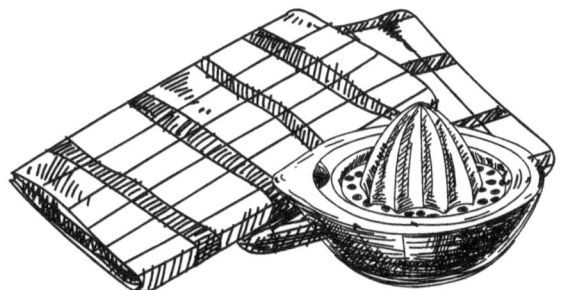

## Great Fruit Choices

Try to eat mostly fresh fruit – limit fruit juice.
Suggested serving size: ½ cup (1 ½ cups daily).

| | | |
|---|---|---|
| Apples | Guava | Oranges |
| Apricots | Jackfruit | Papaya |
| Avocado | Kiwi | Peaches |
| Bananas | Kumquat | Pears |
| Berries | Lemons | Persimmon |
| Cherries | Limes | Pineapple |
| Cranberries | Loquat | Plantains |
| Dates | Mangos | Plums |
| Dragonfruit | Melon (cantaloupe, honeydew, watermelon) | Pomegranate |
| Figs | | Pomelos |
| Grapefruit | | Prunes |
| Grapes | Muscadines | Tangerine |
| | Nectarines | |

# Dairy

This category includes products from cow's milk such as cheese and yogurt, as well as fortified soy milk, soy cheese, soy yogurt, and goat's milk.

Children ages three to eight (3–8) should aim for two cups per day. One and a half ounces of cheese – roughly the size of one piece of string cheese or about ⅓ cup shredded cheese – can be considered equivalent to one cup of milk. Teenagers and adults should aim for three cups of milk (or its equivalent) per day. Choose low-fat sources whenever possible.

Recommended calcium intake for children ages four to eight (4–8) is 800 mg per day. Ages nine to eighteen (9–18) should be getting 1300 mg per day because this is the time in life when bone formation is at its highest point. The school years are a critical time for building strong bones and the most effective time to begin preventing osteoporosis. There is also evidence that calcium intake at recommended levels may correlate with lower body fat. Getting the recommended servings of low-fat dairy is one way to fight childhood obesity.

Items in this category are a great source of several vital nutrients. Most dairy is high in calcium and often fortified with vitamins A and D. In dairy products, these nutrients are packaged in a way that makes them easy for the body to absorb. Other key nutrients include riboflavin, phosphorus, potassium, and magnesium.

Dairy is also high in quality protein. Yogurt has probiotics – tiny microorganisms that are beneficial for the colon and the body's immune system.

## Some suggestions:

- Start with ready-to-eat cereal and ⅔ cup of 1 % milk.

- Enjoy a cup of yogurt as a snack. Watch the sugar content on the food label.

- If your kids refuse to drink regular milk, try soy milk or chocolate/strawberry flavored milk. Keep in mind that the extra sugars count as a sweet too!

- String cheese is super easy to add to a child's lunch bag (keep it cold for good food safety).

## Food Allergies

Some kids may be allergic to a protein in dairy products. This is different from being lactose intolerant. For kids who can't have dairy, it is important that they still get the recommended amount of calcium and vitamin D from soy, leafy green veggies, and fortified orange juice. Other potentially allergenic foods include nuts, eggs, soy, and fish.

Wait to introduce whole milk until after age one (1), eggs until age two (2), and nuts until age three (3). Speaking to a registered dietitian may be helpful for kids with food allergies or a family history of allergies. See the Resources section for tips on how to find a registered dietitian in your area.

## Great Dairy Choices

Remember that a milkshake and a glass of low-fat milk are not the same thing! Dairy products are one of the best ways to ensure kids are getting the nutrients they need for healthy bones, teeth, and many other functions of the body. Choose fat-free or low-fat. Suggested serving size: ⅔ cup (2 cups daily).

| | | |
|---|---|---|
| Almond milk | Frozen yogurt* | Rice milk |
| Buttermilk | Goat's milk | Sour cream* |
| Cheese | Half and half* | Soy milk |
| Coffee creamer* | Ice cream* | Sweetened condensed milk* |
| Cow's milk | Ice milk* | |
| Cream* | Kefir | Whipped cream* |
| Eggnog* | Milkshakes* | |
| Flavored milk | Pudding* | Yogurt |

*Items should be limited or enjoyed in smaller portions.

# Protein

## Protein is said to be the building blocks of our bodies.

Protein is vital for growing bodies to build and repair muscle, as well as to produce hormones and enzymes. Antibodies, which are part of the body's defense against illness, are also made of protein.

This category contains food from animal sources such as meat, fish, eggs, and dairy, but also contains food from non-animal sources such as beans/legumes, soy/tofu, seeds, and nuts. Animal-based foods in this category provide iron, zinc, and vitamin B12, which are important for growing bodies.

Many grains also contain some protein (although not a complete protein), so combining any of the previous foods with grains can provide a good source of protein for your growing kids.

Vegetarian diets for children and adults can be perfectly healthy and provide adequate protein. Sources of protein include a rich variety of soy/tofu, nuts (no nuts until age three), seeds, and grains, which can all be combined to provide a healthy and satisfying menu.

Vegetarian diets that include some dairy and eggs also provide adequate protein and vitamin B12. Vegetarian families will want to make sure their growing kids have iron- and zinc-rich foods.

Protein needs vary greatly. While it is a central part of the diet, excess protein will be converted to fat and stored. Check to see what is right for your kids at www.choosemyplate.gov.

Consuming excess protein (more than the recommended amount by age) or amino acid powders will not make muscles bigger or stronger – only exercise will do that.

## Some suggestions:

- Choose lean meats such as chicken, turkey breast, or lean beef (flank steak, sirloin, and extra-lean ground beef).

- Go for chicken or turkey without the skin. Ground turkey breast is an alternative to high-fat sausage or hamburger.

- Grilling and baking are much healthier ways to cook meat than high-fat frying. Instead of chicken nuggets, serve baked chicken breast.

- Fish can be a great source of nutrients, including essential fatty acids such as Omega-3.

- Serve tacos or burritos with beans and rice for a yummy, inexpensive, high protein/high fiber dinner.

- Beans, seeds, and nuts can all be added to a colorful salad.

- Warm, comforting soups benefit from added beans.

- Soy products have come a long way. Delicious soy sausage, "chicken" patties, and veggie burgers are a hearty but low-fat meal.

- Soups and stir fry can also be made with tofu. Tofu absorbs the flavors it is cooked with, so don't be shy with the herbs and spices when going with soy.

# Great Protein Choices

Go for lean meats and cook with as little added fat as possible. Non-meat items listed here can be a great and inexpensive way to get protein.

Protein needs vary greatly. The Nutrition Tracking Board is averaged for three to eight (3–8) year olds and has 3 – 5 oz equivalents per day.

Suggested serving size: 1 oz meat, 1 egg, 1 Tbsp peanut butter, ½ oz nuts, or ¼ cup dry beans.

## FISH/ SEAFOOD

| | | | | |
|---|---|---|---|---|
| Bass | Cod | Haddock | Salmon | Snapper |
| Bluefish | Crab | Halibut | Sardines | Tilapia |
| Catfish | Flounder | Herring | Scallops | Trout |
| Clams | Grouper | Lobster | Shrimp | Tuna |

## MEAT/POULTRY

| | | | | |
|---|---|---|---|---|
| Beef | Chicken | Eggs | Lamb | Turkey |
| Bison | Duck | Game | Pork | Venison |

## BEANS (LEGUMES)

| | | | | |
|---|---|---|---|---|
| Black | Kidney | Navy | Soybeans/ Edamame | Tofu (low-fat, adaptable) |
| Garbanzo/ Chickpeas | Lentils | Pinto | Soy Nuts | White |
| | Lima | Red | | |

## NUTS & SEEDS (HIGH UNSATURATED FAT CONTENT)

| | | | | |
|---|---|---|---|---|
| Almonds/ Almond butter | Cashew/ Cashew butter | Peanuts/ Peanut butter | Pistachios | sesame butter) |
| Brazil nuts | Coconut | Pecans | Pumpkin seeds | Sunflower seeds |
| | Macadamia nuts | Pine nuts | Sesame seeds (Tahini/ | Walnuts |

## DAIRY

Milk, cheese, cottage cheese, and low-fat yogurt are in both categories – eat and track them depending on where you need them for the day. Remember to incorporate a variety!

# Fats & Oils

**Dietary fat gives flavor and a smooth, delicious texture to foods.**

Not only is some fat good, but we need fat as part of a healthy diet. Vitamins A, D, E, and K need dietary fat to be absorbed properly by the body.

Body fat is your body's form of stored energy. It insulates you from cold and provides a cushion for vital organs. Fat and cholesterol in the diet is very important for infants and toddlers – whole milk is recommended between the ages of one and two (1–2).

Sounds good, right? Well, it's probably not news to you that in the U.S. we consume too much fat and cholesterol. Starting in childhood, eating a healthy diet with the recommended levels of fat can help prevent chronic diseases such as type II diabetes, heart disease, and high cholesterol.

We should aim for about 25–30% of our daily calories from fat, with 10% or less from saturated fat.

## *Classifications of fats:*

### Saturated fats

We want to limit saturated fats in our diets because they contribute to cardiovascular damage and raise blood cholesterol levels (even in kids).

A few examples of foods that contain saturated fats are butter, stick margarine, lard, shortening, sausage, hamburger, bacon and other pork products, processed meats, whole dairy products, ice cream, fried foods, doughnuts, cookies, many baked goods, ranch dressing, hydrogenated oils, coconut oil, and palm oil.

### Trans fats

These raise bad cholesterol and lower good cholesterol. They are found in commercially made baked goods, microwave popcorn, margarine, and foods that are made with partially hydrogenated vegetable oils.

Avoid these as much as possible. Trans fats are listed on the food label.

### Unsaturated fats
### (e.g., mono-unsaturated and polyunsaturated fats)

These fats still have the same amount of calories per gram but are considered healthier for the body. They don't raise bad cholesterol and contain vitamin E. They may decrease total cholesterol if substituted for saturated fats in the diet.

Two good sources of unsaturated fat are olive oil and canola oil. A tablespoon of olive oil can be added instead of butter when cooking rice, couscous, or other grain products. It also makes a flavorful addition to homemade salad dressing.

Canola oil is a good choice because it can tolerate higher cooking temperatures than olive oil and has been shown to reduce total cholesterol when used as a replacement for saturated fats.

Nuts such as almonds, walnuts, and peanuts also provide mostly unsaturated fat, as well as some vitamins, minerals, and protein.

These examples of fat are considered "good" fats, but they are still high in calories. Therefore it is important to watch portion sizes with oils and nuts. For kids ages three to eight (3–8) that means only about four (4) teaspoons of oil or its equivalent per day.

## Essential fatty acids

Essential fatty acids are the omega-3 and omega-6 fats. You may have also heard them called linolenic acid (EPA and DHA) and lenoleic acid.

These are considered essential because the body really needs them but can't make them on its own. You have to get them from food. Omega-6 is actually pretty common in a typical western diet already. Getting enough omega-3 takes a little thought.

Omega-3 fatty acids help the brain function better, may help improve learning and memory, are important for good eye health, have been shown to protect the cardiovascular system, and reduce inflammation.

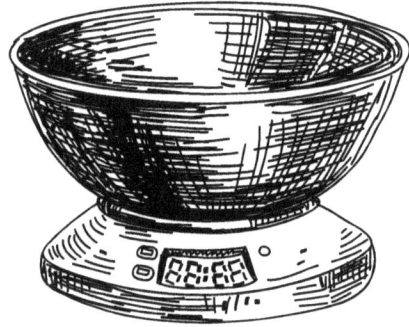

### Where do you find omega-3 fatty acids?

- FISH! All kinds of fish, but especially fatty fish like salmon, herring, sardines, and trout. Varieties of fish that come from cold water contain more omega-3.

- Flax seeds and flax seed oil

- Walnuts

- Canola oil and olive oil

Many products at your grocery store are now fortified with omega-3. It will be listed on the package. Examples are eggs, yogurt, pasta, peanut butter, and cereals.

# Sweets & Extras

**Just because I have a degree in nutrition doesn't mean that I don't need my chocolate sometimes.**

I am also a big fan of Girl Scout cookies! I am a believer in just about anything in moderation.

Have a couple of cookies, just don't have the whole box. Have a candy bar from time to time, just don't have the super size one. Better yet, split something sweet with a friend. Can't imagine life without french fries? That's okay – why not get the kid size on special occasions? These are discretionary calories and extras on the Rule a Healthy Roost Nutrition Tracking Board.

Got cravings? Buy it. Throw away all but a few bites of it immediately. Eat the rest. Really enjoy it. Get on with your day and take the stairs to celebrate!

Soft drink consumption in the U.S. is at an all-time high. Portion sizes of these high-calorie, high-sugar beverages are way too high (20 oz, 32 oz, yikes!).

We call these empty calorie foods because you don't get any other nutrients. Soft drink consumption has been linked to the current epidemic level of childhood obesity. They have also been linked to reduced calcium intake in children and adolescents. Save soft drinks and artificially flavored drinks for special occasions, and drink water and milk at meal times.

Maintaining a healthy weight is really all about energy balance. Energy in the form of food (calories) goes in, and you burn energy as you go about your day and when you exercise. Finding that balance requires watching portion sizes, enjoying a variety of foods, and engaging in physical activity.

Food is a delicious part of a life well lived. Healthy food can be made in wonderful, satisfying ways, and teaching your kids about a healthy lifestyle that includes good food and physical activity is a gift that lasts for generations.

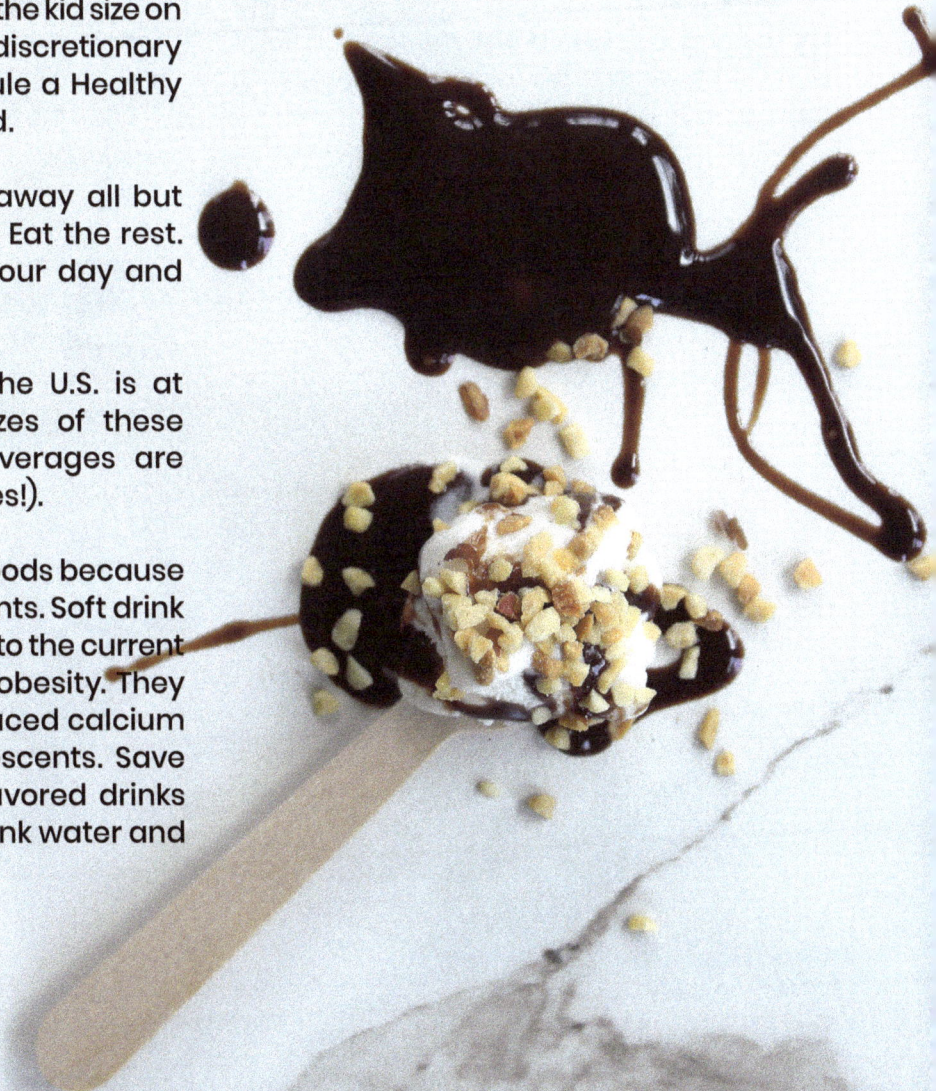

# Snacks

## Snacks are an important part of a healthy diet.

Kids especially need designated snack times. We all know how easy it is to get tired, unmotivated, and grouchy when you are hungry.

Fitting all the important nutrients into three meals a day isn't good for kids (or adults). Dividing up the total daily intake into six meals helps keep blood sugar stable, promotes learning, helps maintain energy levels, and reduces grouchiness. This may be tricky with kids in school. You might try tossing a granola bar, piece of fruit, or peanut butter sandwich into their book bag for the 10:00 am or after-school snack.

## *Healthy Ways to Snack*

- VEGGIES! If they are washed, cut, and ready to eat, they will more likely be eaten. Try to have fresh veggies cut into snack-sized pieces in the fridge: carrots, celery, colorful peppers (red, orange, yellow, green), cucumbers, or tiny tomatoes.

- Talk to your child's teachers about their snack time at school and what foods are appropriate for them to bring.

- If snacks are provided by the school, ask what they are, and if they aren't appropriate, find a nice way to talk to the school about it. Oreo cookies aren't an appropriate snack to have each day!

- If parents provide snacks, then try to help your teachers put together a good list of healthy snacks that they can give to parents. Lack of refrigeration will likely be an issue – try to come up with healthy extended shelf-life snacks (pretzels, whole wheat snack crackers, graham crackers, cheese whiz – kiddin'!).

- Try to bring fresh fruit for your child's class when you can.

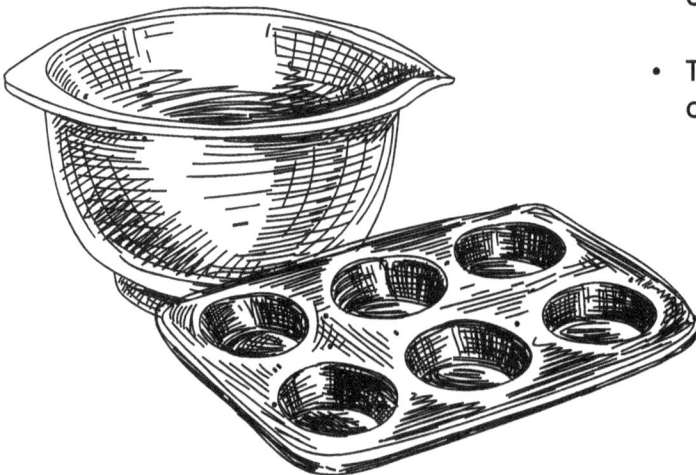

# Kitchen

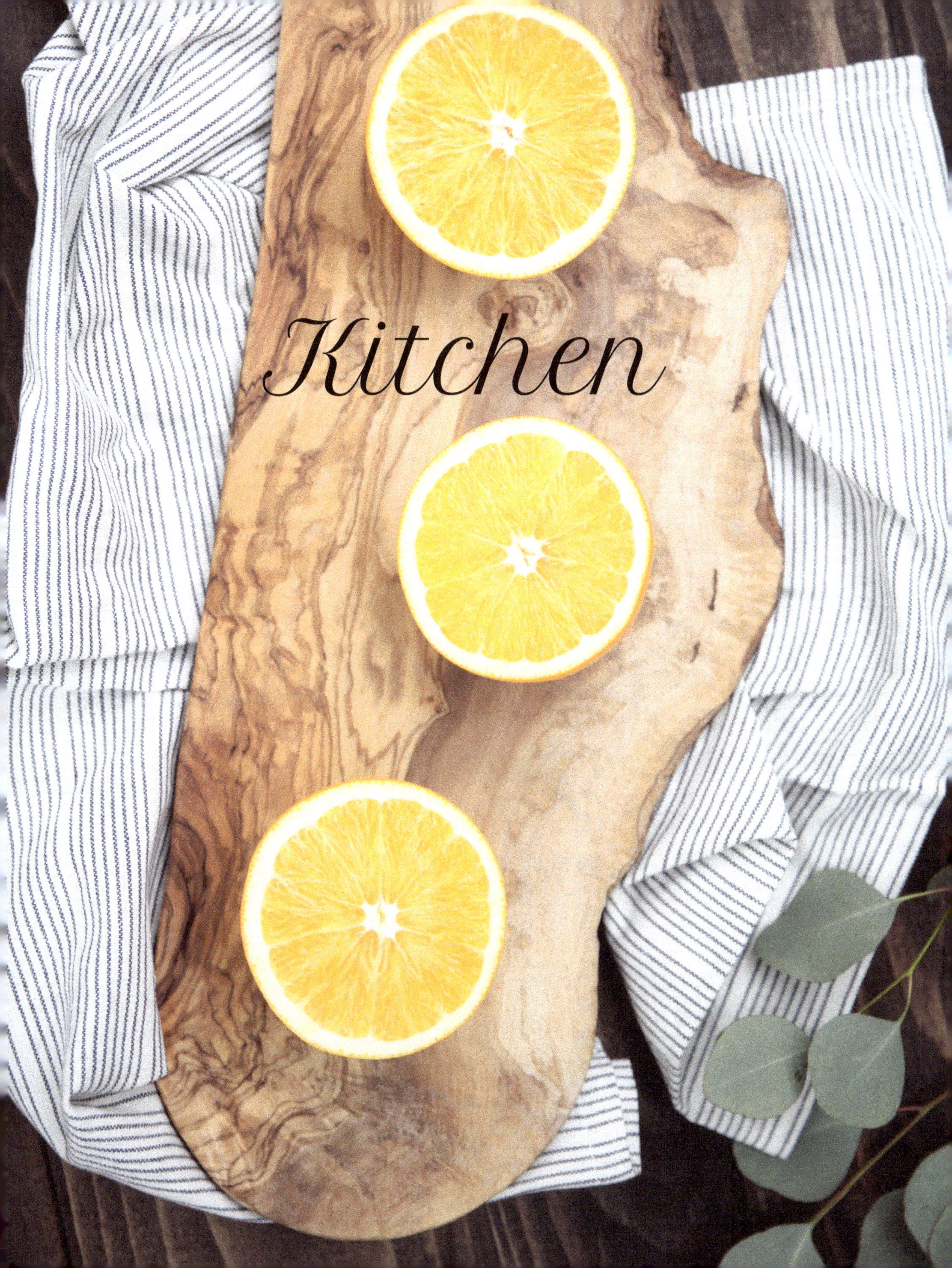

# Building a Nutritious Kitchen

In this section, we gathered some tips and good advice that will help you lay out a nutritious kitchen. If you have fresh nutritious foods, the proper tools to prepare them, and are organized about food choices, you'll increase your chances of eating better. I've found that the times we eat the worst are when we don't have healthy choices readily available. Convenience has become the way of the world, especially with families getting busier each day.

If you find yourself getting a meal at a convenience store, you might want to take a step back and re-evaluate. By organizing your "food life" a little better, it'll be much simpler to eat well and not live with a bunch of last-minute decisions sitting around your waist and on your conscience.

We asked a wide range of folks to help us pass along their traditions and knowledge. You will find tips from our community in the back of this section. Thanks to members of the Grant Park Parent Network, Grant Park Cooperative Preschool, and all the other folks who contributed ideas!

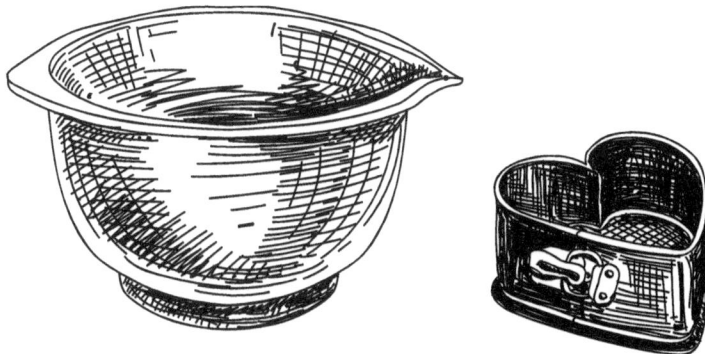

# Volume Equivalents

| Fluid Ounce | Teaspoon | Tablespoon | Cup | Pint | Quart | Gallon |
|---|---|---|---|---|---|---|
| | 3 tsp. | 1 Tbsp. | | | | |
| | | 4 Tbsp. | 1/4 cup | | | |
| 4 oz. | | 8 Tbsp. | 1/2 cup | | | |
| 8 oz. | | 16 Tbsp. | 1 cup | 1/2 pint | | |
| 16 oz. | | | 2 cups | 1 pint | | |
| | | | 4 cups | 2 pints | 1 quart | |
| | | | 8 cups | 4 pints | 2 quarts | 1/2 gallon |
| | | | 16 cups | 8 pints | 4 quarts | 1 gallon |

## Weight Equivalent:

1 pound = 16 ounces

# Emergency Substitutions

| Need | Substitute |
|---|---|
| Shallots | White onion or white part of scallions |
| Eggs (1 large) | 2 egg whites |
| Lemon juice | White vinegar or lime juice |
| Buttermilk (1 cup) | 1 cup plain low-fat yogurt or 1 cup minus 1 tablespoon milk + 1 tablespoon lemon juice or white vinegar |
| Cottage cheese | Ricotta cheese |
| Sour cream | Plain yogurt |
| Cream, heavy | Whipping cream |
| Crème Fraiche (1 cup) | ½ cup sour cream + ½ cup heavy cream |
| Chocolate, semisweet (1 oz) | 1 oz bittersweet or 1 oz unsweetened chocolate + 1 tablespoon sugar |
| Breadcrumbs | Crushed crackers, panko, matzo meal, or cornflakes |
| Herbs, fresh chopped (1 tablespoon) | 1 teaspoon dried herbs |
| Poultry seasoning (1 teaspoon) | ¾ teaspoon ground sage + ¼ teaspoon ground thyme |
| Pumpkin pie spice (1 teaspoon) | ½ teaspoon ground cinnamon + ¼ teaspoon ground ginger + ⅛ teaspoon ground nutmeg + ⅛ teaspoon ground cloves |
| Baking powder (1 teaspoon) | ¼ teaspoon baking soda + ½ teaspoon cream of tartar |
| Cornstarch (1 tablespoon) | 2 tablespoons flour or 4 teaspoons quick-cooking tapioca |

# Pantry Tips

## Keep it shallow!

If you have a shallow pantry, you might be less likely to overbuy and let food go bad. The theory is that if you can see it, you will use it. I know one family (no names!) that had four bags of flour, twelve boxes of cereal, twelve cans of veg-all, a sticky jar of molasses (don't ask), and over twenty cans of food (not including the veg-all) that all had expired over the last year or two. Not only is this a great waste of money, but eww!

## *Some suggestions:*

- If you have a deep pantry without those fancy pull-out shelves, try this trick. Get some shoe boxes. Paint or wrap them in pretty paper just for fun, and put them in the back of the pantry. They will prevent your food from falling into the "land of no return."

- Try to turn over the contents of your pantry at least every three months to make sure you are using what you have. Check expiration dates and look for signs of "friends" that have come to visit. Keep flour and other grains in sealed containers and preferably in the fridge (keeps it fresher and critters don't like the cold).

- Make sure your pantry is well ventilated and stays cool.

If you have foods you'd like your kids to snack on, put them
in their line of sight and within their reach.

Prepare portioned servings of snacks like crackers, pretzels, etc., so they
can take a serving size rather than the whole bag. Cut up veggies and
cheese and place in individual serving containers in the fridge.

Have a designated place for their snacks. Make sure
it's easy to grab a healthy snack!

# Refrigerator Organization

## Shallow fridge!

Nothing is so precious or durable that it needs to stay in your refrigerator more than a few months (sauces, etc., can hang around for a while – check the dates).

Know what is in your fridge and use it often. Go through your supply of food and try not to overbuy. Your refrigerator actually needs air to circulate to keep foods their freshest.

If you need sour cream for the week ahead and you are at the grocery store, you should buy some more. If you get home and find you have four unopened containers of sour cream in the fridge, you should reevaluate your organization and shopping list techniques.

If you constantly find mystery items at the back of your fridge, then try to get rid of the back of your fridge. Get some large containers and fill them with water (or store your flour in them!). They will prevent foods from getting lost in the back. Added bonus: liquids/solids hold the cold better than air, so each time you open the fridge you will get a little jingle in your pocket (well, not literally).

If you have developed a personal relationship with anything in your fridge, you might need to let it go. I did have a jar of pickles my mother made in my fridge for five years. She had prepared them for Christmas dinner, and it was the last thing she made for me before she suddenly passed away. It took me a while to "detach."

## *How to organize your fridge:*

- Cooked foods go on the top shelf.

- Dairy goes on the next shelf.

- Deli meats and cheese can be stored in the drawer, but don't place raw meats in the drawer with them!

- Veggies must be separate from raw and cooked proteins.

- Anything in the door will be exposed to the greatest temperature changes. It's not the ideal place for milk and eggs if you open and close your fridge a lot.

- Any raw food must be in a pan at the very bottom, with no cooked foods underneath it.

# Basic Food Safety

Food safety is really about not making you or your family sick. No one likes an upset tummy after eating mom's cooking. (My friend's mother eats expired food all the time and refrigerates things she's cooked right in the pot, with the spoon still in it. She is not a child, has a cast iron stomach, and can get away with this behavior. Do not try this at home!)

A foodborne illness is a disease that is carried or transmitted to people by food. Most foodborne illnesses are caused by microorganisms such as bacteria, viruses, parasites, and fungi.

Once bacteria has been transmitted onto food, it can grow rapidly under conditions such as high moisture, high protein, and low acidity.

## Food can become unsafe in four ways:

1. **Poor Personal Hygiene**
   Not washing hands properly, not covering cuts, touching body parts, and wearing jewelry (take your rings off) are all examples of poor hygiene in the kitchen.

2. **Cross-Contamination**
   This term describes the transfer of microorganisms from one food or surface to another.

   Cross-contamination is caused by not washing hands, improper cleaning and sanitizing, surfaces and utensils touching both raw and ready-to-eat foods, and improperly storing raw foods over ready-to-eat foods.

3. **Time-Temperature Abuse**
   Food that is allowed to remain in the temperature danger zone (40–140°F) can become potentially hazardous by allowing bacteria to multiply. Keeping hot foods hot and cold foods cold can prevent time-temperature abuse.

4. **Improper Cleaning and Sanitizing**
   Foods are contaminated when they come into contact with surfaces that are not cleaned and sanitized regularly.

## How to prevent cross-contamination
### Two words: clean and sanitize

Cleaning removes visible signs of soil, while sanitizing removes harmful levels of bacterial contamination. But be really careful mixing chemicals!

## Steps to take

1. **KEEP UP WITH YOUR FRIDGE!**

- The temperature inside should always be below 40°F (use a thermometer to check).

- Wipe up spills immediately and clean surfaces thoroughly with hot, soapy water, then rinse.

- Refrigerate or freeze meat and poultry the minute you're home from the store.

- Keep the door closed as much as possible, and don't store perishable stuff like milk or eggs in the door.

## 2. THAW CORRECTLY

- Freezing prevents bacteria from multiplying but does not kill it. Bacteria can and will multiply as food begins to thaw.

- Thaw food in the refrigerator at 41°F or less.

- Thaw food by submerging it under running, drinkable water that is 70°F or less.

- Thaw food as part of the cooking process.

- Thaw food in the microwave only if the food will be cooked immediately.

## 3. COOK IT UP RIGHT

- Know the minimum internal cooking temperatures required for various foods.

- **Watch out for the 100 Degrees of Doom.** Food (raw and cooked) can become unsafe if it dwells anywhere between 40°F and 140°F. So keep your fridge set to 37°F and make sure your cooked food hits above 140°F.

- **Meat Temperature Doneness**

  **140°F** – Rare beef, ham
  (pre-cooked)
  **145°F** – Medium rare beef, lamb
  **160°F** – Medium beef, veal, lamb,
  ham (raw)
  **170°F** – Well-done beef, pork,
  veal, lamb
  **180°F** – Chicken and turkey
  (whole)

## 4. MANAGE YOUR LEFTOVERS

- Make it a weekly habit to throw out expired foods that should no longer be eaten.

- Divide leftovers into small portions and store in shallow, tightly sealed containers (two inches deep or less).

- Date leftovers so you know how long they've been in the refrigerator. As a general rule of thumb, discard cooked leftovers after four days.

- Remember the two-hour rule for refrigeration. Perishable leftovers from a meal should not stay out of refrigeration for more than two hours. In hot weather (90°F or above) this time is reduced to one hour.

**When in doubt, throw it out!**

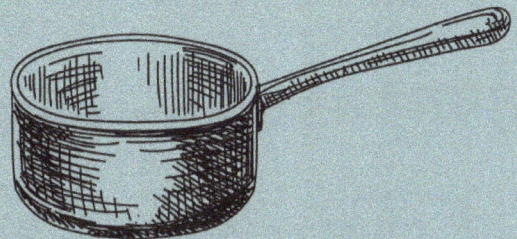

# Kitchen Safety Tips

## Discuss with your kids!

Safety should always be your first priority! The most important tip you need to teach your children is that they need to follow certain rules in the kitchen.

You certainly don't want them to grow up afraid of the kitchen. Learning some basic rules should help them stay happy and hurt-free in the kitchen.

## At the Stove

- Always be sure a responsible adult or older child is paying attention the entire time the stove is on, especially when using gas burner stoves with an open flame!

- Always have a fire extinguisher on hand, and make sure your older children know where it is and how to use it.

- Do not place any easily incendiary items (like placemats, dish towels, paper towels, etc.) next to the stove! They could shift into the flame and start a quick and deadly fire.

- Always make sure you have snug-fitting clothes – shirttails and sleeves should be out of the way. Wear an apron – it will keep mess to a minimum and hold your clothes away from the flames.

- Tie back long hair.

- Always turn pot handles to the inside/middle of the stove. One brush with an arm could be remembered for a lifetime.

- Get child-proof caps to go over the controls on your stove until your kids are old enough to use it independently.

- Make sure your stove will not tip over! There are anti-tip devices you can install. Never let your child sit, stand, or crawl on the open door of the oven.

You think it wouldn't happen but I've found my son up there. Fortunately the oven wasn't on. Our bedtime story that night was "Hansel and Gretel."

## Dishwasher

- Always load knives with the points down or laying flat in the rack.

- Never stand on the open dishwasher door. No matter what your kids say about needing to reach something, they don't have enough allowance to replace the hinges.

## Fridge

- Never get in it! It's cold, and you can't breathe after a while.

- Don't hang on the doors while they are open or the door handles while closed. The refrigerator could tip over, or the door handles could fall off – they don't have enough allowance to pay for that either!

## Small Appliances

- Keep small appliances unplugged when not in use. Paper towels will "toast" and catch on fire.

# Kids in the Kitchen

## Train Them Up Right!

Children should learn at an appropriate age how to use different common kitchen utensils. Try them on the veggie/potato peeler and cheese shredder at about five years old. (You might need some band-aids and a year or two.)

About eight or nine years old should be a good age to let them try to use the knives. (You know best when to encourage this. Just make sure you do let them take charge at some point.)

Make sure you have a good set of knives and that they stay sharp (they cut better and are less likely to result in an accident). Teach kids to curl their fingertips under when they are holding food down on the cutting board.

There is no need for speed – safety is the priority!

## *Some suggestions:*

- Spend a night or two watching a cooking show on TV and pay attention to the chef's technique – talk about it with your kids.

- Take a cooking class with your kids. (Check out this mom-preneur business, Young Chef's Academy, at: www.youngchefsacademy.com.)

- Don't be discouraged if you get many different sizes (the goal is to have equally sized foods if they are to be cooked so the cooking time evens out). Always encourage the act rather than the final product.

## The Magic of Mise en Place

How many times have you seen a cooking show and they always start with perfectly chopped ingredients in little pre-measured cups? Somebody had to chop all that food at some point, and it wasn't an elf or a brownie.

Gather the ingredients before you start cooking, and then have a good time with your prep work. Turn on some good music and have a weekly chopping party! If you know your weekly menu and can plan ahead what you need to chop, it will cut down on your daily need to prep for each meal.

This is a great time to cut up some extra veggies for snacking during the week. Nothing is better than being hungry and having some celery and red pepper chopped and ready to go! Instant satisfaction, and no guilt to boot.

# Kitchen Equipment

## *Good Knives*

Invest in good knives – they'll last a lifetime. Having quality knives, and knowing how to use and sharpen them, will change your enthusiasm for food prep. Don't have a lot of money? Just buy one at a time. You really only need three types of knives, so buying them one at a time is practical. Avoid the big knife blocks – you might not need all the knives that come with it.

You do need: a chef's knife, a paring knife (or two), and a serrated (bumpy edge) knife for cutting bread. A carving knife is nice, but the chef's knife will do the job.

## *A Cutting Board or Two or Three*

Get a few, and clearly mark one for cutting raw meat and poultry. The one you use for cutting raw meat should not be made of wood – plastic works best, but look for one that won't dull those fancy knives you've been saving up for (acrylic boards are famous for being knife killers).

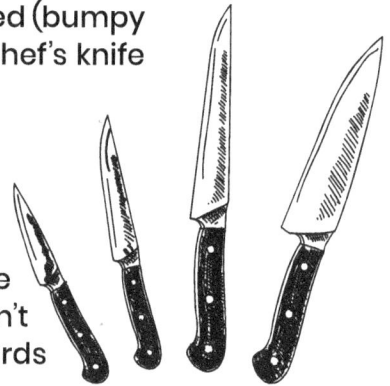

You do not want your raw veggies chopped on the same board that had poultry juice on it the day before. Can you say salmonella? Can you spell botulism?

## *Pressure Cooker/Instapot*

Do you have memories of those old-fashioned pressure cookers your grandma used to use? The ones that were made of aluminum and sounded like an airplane taking off? Scary stuff, those – never knew when they were going to blow.

Well, revise your thinking. American cooks are among the only ones in the world who don't regularly use pressure cookers, and it's our loss. Modern pressure cookers have great safety features, are made of stainless steel, sleekly designed, and have a functionality that will make cooking take about 70% less time than conventional methods. Pressure cookers work by sealing and locking. Pressure then builds inside the pot, and the resulting steam infuses the flavors and cooks the food quickly.

A strong word of caution: If you have inherited one of those old pressure cookers, or come across one at a yard sale, do yourself a huge favor and either throw it out or use it to water your plants. The seals on those old cookers can fail, and they just weren't safe. Aluminum is a poor choice for cookware as it can pit and develop cracks.

# Cast Iron

Cast iron is an excellent heat conductor. A properly seasoned cast iron pan can last for generations and, best of all, is practically non-stick. Unlike non-stick skillets, cast iron can go straight from the cooktop to the oven.

Cast iron pans are very inexpensive – a good brand is Lodge, and they now offer pre-seasoned pans, most under $30. Every kitchen should have a Dutch oven and a 10" and a 12" skillet – once you have that big 12" skillet, you'll be amazed you ever did without it.

Keeping up with seasoning is super simple. After cleaning the pan (I clean mine with a nylon scrubber and a little dish detergent – a well-seasoned pan can handle water and detergent) dry it out with a towel, and put it back on the burner to heat up little. Once the pan is warm, take it off the burner, spray it with vegetable cooking spray, and then wipe it down with a paper towel.

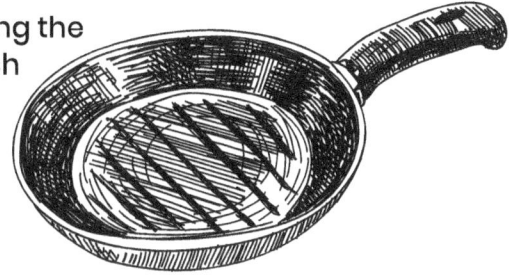

# Non-stick Skillet

If you don't have cast iron, then you need at least one medium non-stick skillet. Just be sure to not use metal utensils. Non-stick cookware has to be disposed of when the coating begins to deteriorate. There is a more "healthy" version of non-stick cookware available these days – check out the GreenPan™.

# Saucepans

Most kitchens will only ever need two saucepans – a small one and a large one (1.5 quart and 4 quart). A medium sauce pan can also come in handy, so look for 2.5 and 3 quart options.

For the small one, look for one with a pour spout – very handy for delicate sauces which need to be removed from the pan quickly. The medium saucepan should have a tight-fitting lid and be heavy enough to conduct heat.

The very best saucepans are made of copper with a tin lining, but those cost big bucks. Unless you are really into cooking and can afford it, a saucepan made of stainless steel with an aluminum or copper core is very versatile, and you can find one in any price range. Another option is hard, anodized aluminum, but those are not dishwasher safe. For a large saucepan, look for a stay-cool handle and a side helper handle.

**Note about aluminum cookware:** Do not use regular aluminum pots for cooking acidic foods (tomato sauce, etc.) or green veggies – bad interaction, 'nuff said.

# Slow Cooker/Crock Pot

The original put-it-in-and-forget-about-it wonder of the kitchen. Slow cookers can make even the toughest cut of meat tender and delicious. Look for a slow cooker with a warm option – very handy for serving spiced wine at the holidays. Another nice feature is a removable insert. This allows you to put everything together the night before and refrigerate. Just be sure to bring to room temperature before putting it in the base.

# Strainer vs. Colander vs. Sieve

They are all designed to do the same thing – strain food – but each is slightly different and used for different purposes. A colander has feet and is used to simply drain something. It has large holes and handles. A sieve usually does not have feet since it's placed over another bowl. A sieve is made of fine mesh and can be used to strain foods that need a fine texture – for instance, to strain seeds out of a sauce or lumps out of gravy. Both are sometimes called strainers, which is where it gets confusing.

You need one of each. A large colander is more useful than a small one, and a smaller sieve is more useful than a too-large one. So, big colander, small sieve.

## Peelers

Children love to peel things. Buy nice peelers with sturdy handles, and make sure you have one per child.

## Graters

Older children can use a micro hand grater to help. The old box graters are harder for them to operate. Have your kids grate onto a paper towel – the texture of the paper towel will help keep the grater from slipping.

Hand graters come in a variety of styles to suit different types of grating tasks. Because they are small, they fit easily into drawers. Look for the kind that have a thick handle. That makes them easier for small hands to grip.

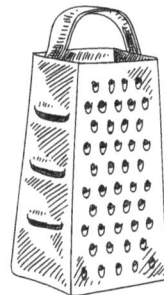

## Plasticware

Try to get the kind where every size uses the same size lids. Square fits better in the fridge. Buy lots that are small in size, and you can use them for packing lunches and eliminate all the little plastic baggies.

**DON'T use plastic in the microwave!** Purchase some glass storage containers, and always use microwave-safe containers to heat food. Stay away from plastics and plastic wrap, especially when microwaving.

# At the Table

## Place Setting

Have your kids draw their place setting on a piece of paper (10" x 15" or so) and laminate it. Teach them why we eat with utensils (it separates us from the animals), why the ones we have are used, and why they are placed where they are.

Did you know that if you hold your hands straight out and make a circle with your thumb and forefinger on each hand, the left will form a lowercase "b" and the right will form a lower case "d." Just remember "b"read – LEFT and "d"rink – RIGHT.

## Placemats

We use fun laminated placemats. (The kids can make their own, and you can have them laminated at your local copy shop.) They are a heck of a lot easier to clean than a tablecloth. Just dump off the remnants of your feeding frenzy and rinse in the sink.

I have a bad habit of letting them sit on the side of the sink to "dry." They never do – they just end up damp and stuck together. Instead, roll them up on top of a dishtowel (like a jellyroll) and they are ready to go again!

## Try the European Method

Did you know that the reason you turn your knife and fork toward your plate is because the knife used to serve not only as an eating utensil, but also as your weapon? That's why we have such strong rules about pointing your utensils at your dining partners.

The fork was a Middle Eastern invention of the 11th century, but did not come into common use in England until 1608. Because America was already colonized, we got our forks a little later, so we have a different eating style than most of the Western world. Our style of eating (cutting with the dominant hand, then switching the fork to the dominant hand and putting the knife down) is called the Zig Zag Method.

We've grown rather attached to our style of eating, but if you think about it, the European style (where the fork lives in the left hand and the knife lives in the right) actually makes quite a bit of sense. In the European Method, your fork is held with the tines down, toward your plate, and your knife acts as a helper to stabilize food as you push it onto the down tines of the fork. So much easier! You can "stab" your food – gently of course, and using nice manners, no self-defense maneuvers that would make a Viking proud – so that even the most difficult morsels make it easily onto the fork.

If you eat using the European Method, you don't have those pesky elbows waving around in the air. If your kids are like mine, you'll also find they naturally have better posture using this method – and we all know posture is important to digestion. And the best part? Table setting will once again make sense because the positions of the knife and fork relate to how they are actually used.

## Table Manners

### Teach your kids good table manners early on. You'll never regret it.

If there is more expectation of your kids helping set the table and serve dinner, and more talk about why you eat what you do, then dinner might be more fun for everyone. Removing their plates, scraping them, and putting them in the dishwasher is a respectful habit to teach at an early age.

Want more polished kids? Search for an etiquette class in your area!

**A tip about manners from our friend Lucia:**

Just as important as teaching our children the right kinds and right amounts of foods they need each day is helping them develop good manners – especially when eating. To be prepared for life, we all need to know the proper way to behave, and it is our responsibility as parents to help our children prepare to be adults – adults who have good attitudes, as well as respect and consideration for others at all times.

If children begin with a simple "please" and "thank you" when they are very young, they will build a strong foundation on their way to being well-mannered people. The more children repeat good etiquette practices, the more these practices will become a natural extension of themselves. Raising a well-mannered child begins at home, at the dinner table, as a family.

– Lucia C. Johnson
The Life Lessons Academy, Rome, GA

### Would you like a little whine with your dinner?

Ever heard this one? "How many more bites do I have to eat?" I thought so. Try this response: "I don't know. Why don't you count them and let me know when you are done?" If it works, let us know!

It is up to you what to do about "I'm done, can I get up?" You as a parent have to decide if they are to remain at the table until everyone is done or if they may quietly excuse themselves when they are done. Figure out what is right for your family, and try to balance it with your child's attention, physical abilities for their age, and the absolute right of everyone to eat a meal in peace.

Let your children help you put the food on their plates, and explain why they need to eat the different foods as you go. (Brush up on the nutritional info and what different foods do in the previous section, Nutrition.)

**And remember: You are not their short order cook.** Talk to your family beforehand about what you are cooking, and if you choose to offer choices, make them equal. "We are having salad, chicken, and rice for dinner." If you get an "I hate salad" response, then try to follow up with something like: "You can have the parts of the salad separate or just some carrot sticks." Try at all costs not to revert to the "Well, what would you like then?" response. You will end up listing everything in the fridge, pantry, and grocery store before you find "something they want."

Get them on board – let them know which little markers they will be able to move after dinner with the meal you have prepared.

**Don't be rude – eat your food.** The idea that you need to eat everything on your plate in order to be "polite" should be examined. Children should be encouraged to try everything they are served, especially at someone else's home, but let's face it – do you really want your child yacking up on someone's tablecloth because they really can't stand what is on their plate?

Many times they are being dramatic (see later chapter on how to be dramatic in a good way) but they may really have an aversion to their friend's favorite family recipe – squash and lima bean casserole. Teach them to politely ask that they be excused from eating something.

**Be careful about the "clean plate club" as well.** Most likely this idea developed in a time when food was a much more precious resource that "shouldn't be wasted" because you didn't know where your next meal was coming from. "It took yer daddy three days to trap that. Now stop fussin' and eat!" (If daddy really did spend three days trapping it, then they probably will scarf it up). Serve healthy portion sizes and try not to obsess about them finishing every bite. (See Food as Reward in the next section.)

> Remember: You don't serve wine to your children,
> and they in turn shouldn't serve whine to you.

# Food Value

## *Food as Reward*

Many times sweets will be used as a reward: "If you eat all of your veggies you can have dessert." What they will hear after a while is "sweets are a better food, and you can only get them if you eat or do something you don't like." This is setting you up for a world of trouble.

The reason we prioritize sweets as "after you've eaten your veggies" should be explained in a way that they can understand. Use your Nutrition Tracking Board to show them what their bodies need to eat each day to grow strong, and once they take care of building strong bodies, they can fill the little bit of room they have left with a moderate-sized treat.

Try to serve sweets and treats on weekends only, or devise some other system that works for your family, so they are not expected after every meal, every day. Do they want a soda? Fine, just drink a little glass of water first!

Do not give a child dessert in order to make them behave! (Oh, can't you just hear that can of worms being popped open?)

## *Where is the Value in Value Menus?*

Food these days is relatively inexpensive and plentiful – too plentiful in many cases. Value menus encourage overeating by the tons each year, for only $1.00 an item! What a bargain.

Teach your children what it really means to value something – that they should place more value on the quality of the food they put in their bodies than the dollars in their wallet. Value real foods and their purpose – to nourish our bodies. Value does not mean being processed to the ends of the earth, shipped, served in ridiculous portions, and sold for only a dollar!

OK, off the soapbox temporarily. I realize that there isn't a family on the block that isn't going to hit the drive-thru from time to time. Just make good choices when you do. Encourage healthy choices no matter how unhealthy the restaurant is overall. Try to spend a little extra if your child wants to opt for the salad option, even though the kid's meal is two dollars less.

Be careful about how much food you serve to your kids and the value that you place on it. It is absolutely OK to throw away half an order of french fries or half a large soda to control their portion sizes.

We don't want to encourage children to waste anything - but if they are served three portions of soda, do you really need them to press on and drink it all because you paid a dollar for it? They should be taught where food comes from (not the grocery store, but before that) and why we have so much of it when other countries do not.

# A Sample Six-Meal Day

### 7:30 AM BREAKFAST

Grain, calcium/dairy, protein, fruit

### 10:00 AM SNACK

Fruit, calcium/dairy (can swap with PM snack)

### 12:00 LUNCH

Grain, grain, veggie, calcium/dairy, protein

### 3:00 PM SNACK

Veggie, grain (can swap with AM snack)

### 6:00 PM DINNER

Grain, veggie, veggie, protein

### 8:00 PM DESSERT

Fruit

## Talk About Your Mouthfuls

Have frequent, rational conversations with your children about food. Teach them to respect food (that it is worthy of respect) and their bodies.

Try to teach your children about good foods – why some actually nourish their bodies and others make them unhealthy. Let them know that they should stop eating those good foods when they are full. Hunger should be the guiding principle for how much to eat – not guilt or social propriety.

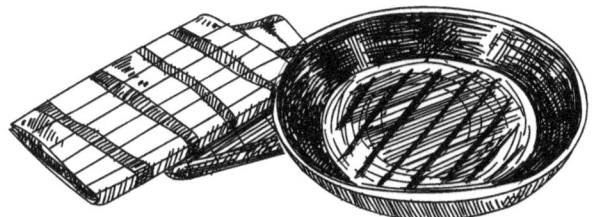

# Portion Control

Serve your children healthy amounts of food. It is probably less than what we are accustomed to in our society. If they have skipped something earlier in the day, don't try to make up for it by serving double portions. Their bellies are only so big.

If they are used to eating whatever is put in front of them, try to get them into the habit of paying attention to what they need to eat! Just because they are served a huge plate of food does not mean they should eat it all.

Let them help you portion out their own food. Buy some small containers (½ – 1 cup) and mark them so your kids can relate to how much a serving size really is! Make sure to check out www.choosemyplate.gov periodically to adjust the serving sizes for their growing bodies.

There is a trend for companies to package snack foods in 100 calorie packs. This theoretically controls the portion size, but it really increases the amount of packaging and doesn't teach anything about controlling intake. If they work for your family, great. Just be careful that they don't get identified as "healthy" – after all, they are still just snack crackers, and it is easy to keep eating them.

## Free Refills!

If you are eating out and your children are offered refills, politely ask for a water refill instead.

## Read Labels

A serving of juice is NOT a 16 oz bottle! There are at least two servings in most "single" containers.

**Here are a few ways to visualize approximate portions:**

- One adult clenched fist: this is about 8 oz of beverage (more than the ⅔ cup on the Nutrition Tracking Board!) – less than a can of soda! Certainly less than a plastic bottle (16–20 oz or more) from a drink machine.

- One adult hand cupped: this is about ½ cup of rice, pasta, fruit, etc.

- Two adult hands cupped: about 1 cup of salad, cereal, etc.

- The palm of one adult hand, or a deck of cards: about 3 oz of cooked meat.

- Two thumbs put together: about one tablespoon.

# Kitchen Tips
*from Our Tables to Yours*

We've put together a short compendium of hand-me-down knowledge – the best kind.

Thanks to all the folks in our community that contributed their tips:

Stephanie, Atlanta, GA | Mama Leslie, Decatur, GA | Janis, Cumming, GA | Mary, Cumming, GA | Ashley, Decatur, GA | Stacy, Atlanta, GA | Laura, Richmond, VA | Michael, Atlanta, GA | Katie, Wadsworth, Ohio | Nichole, Fayetteville, GA | Jennifer P., Atlanta, GA.

**Note:** We have not tested every one of these to make sure they work all of the time. Use your best mom-sense!

- For my "banana pudding" recipe, I use low-fat Banilla yogurt (which they thought for the longest time was actual banana pudding), layer with fresh cut bananas, and top with a homemade whipped cream (which I make with half and half, a bit of honey or raw sugar, and "color" it by blending in some raspberries). Add sliced almonds on top for crunch.

- Dark chocolate is not only yummy, it is also rich in antioxidants.

- You can hide a truck in lasagna. Cook all the veggies you want into the sauce and layer away! Get your eggs in there too with the ricotta cheese/parmesan mixture. No need to cook the noodles beforehand, just make sure they are all touching the sauce.

- Beef and chicken broth together give more flavor to rice, green beans, etc. – use instead of water.

- I like to add roasted winter squash to mac and cheese and quesadillas. Super sweet and it goes unnoticed.

- I chop fresh spinach and toss it in with scrambled eggs and cheese. The spinach wilts quickly, and my kids don't even realize they're eating greens.

- Pop some spinach leaves in the blender with a blueberry smoothie. It hides the color a bit. Tell them it is dinosaur puke!

- Replace half of the white flour in a recipe with whole wheat flour when baking. It has more protein and fiber.

- Peel a banana from the bottom and you won't have to pick the little "stringy things" off of it. That's how primates do it! And take your bananas apart when you get home from the store. If you leave them connected at the stem, they ripen faster.

- Peppers with 3 bumps on the bottom are sweeter and better for eating raw. Peppers with 4 bumps on the bottom are firmer and better for cooking.

- Salt water for pasta after it comes to a boil. It will take longer for the water to boil if you add the salt first.

- If you find that you have over-salted any liquid-based food (i.e., soup, sauce), just add a raw, cut-up baking potato to the mixture while cooking. The potato will absorb the excess salt. Remove the potato before serving.

- Add a teaspoon of water when frying ground beef. It will help to pull the grease away from the meat while cooking. (You still need to get the excess grease out of the pan – be careful!)

- When cutting an onion, leave the root end on. It will help limit tears and give you something to hold on to.

- If you are only using ½ an avocado, leave the pit in the other half. It won't brown as fast with the pit in it.

- Most fresh herbs last longer if you wrap them in a damp paper towel and store in a ziplock bag. Alternatively, put them in water like cut flowers.

- Glass and dark metal baking pans brown more than light metal ones.

- If you remove a skillet from the oven, wrap a dish towel around the handle so you don't forget it's hot. (Make sure not to leave it near the stovetop!)

- I always take my rings off when I cook or clean and then can't remember where I put them. I saw someone using a small elephant statue in their kitchen to hold their rings, so I stole the idea! It's a great help and looks classy too!

- If you're in the grocery store and can't decide what to have for dinner, just look at the pictures on the boxes of frozen dinners for ideas.

- When shopping for whole grains, look for 100% whole grain, not just multigrain.

- Store natural peanut butter upside down. That way, the oil isn't on top.

- Make a fruit and veggie wash from ⅓ part distilled vinegar and 1 part water, and store it in a spray bottle. Spray apples, pears, and other foods that you don't skin before you eat.

- My son likes to help add the spices when I am cooking. Usually if he has helped make the dish, then he will want to eat it.

- Eat locally produced foods. You are not only giving back to your community, your food will be fresher because it usually comes directly from the farm. (Visit www.localharvest.com.)

- Empower your kids. Letting them do tasks for themselves and choose from options you've already deemed acceptable sends the message that you respect them and that you think they are fully capable of accomplishing goals on their own. Simple ideas like hanging a coat rack at their height, putting foods and drinks they are allowed to choose at their level, explaining expectations in advance, and giving them responsibilities that apply to their lives will go a long way toward fortifying their inner confidence and building self-respect. The added benefit is that you are teaching them to think for themselves and guiding them in the direction of fruitful decisions. You only hold the reins for a while.

# Recipes

# Food at the Heart

We simply couldn't do this book without giving you some tasty, tasty recipes. We hope you will enjoy making them with your kids.

Our recipes come from Chef Sheri Davis, who closed her award-winning Atlanta restaurant, Dish, to spend more time with her two growing boys, and then started an incredibly successful catering business called Fresh World Cuisine with her talented husband Vando. You can often find her cooking for her sons and their friends in the local skateboard club. Sheri knows how to feed growing children. Growing up, her family garden gave her the inspiration to train as a chef, so fresh ingredients are always on the menu at Sheri's house. We feel very fortunate to have had the planets align and put Sheri into our path.

> "So, what about the food? Food is at the heart of everything we do to make our kids grow up strong and healthy. Achieving a well-balanced meal does not have to be rocket science. A meal is a marriage – everything on the plate needs to go together and harmonize; the colors must complement, the textures must entice, and the flavors must please. You don't want a whole brown plate or a plate where everything is all mushy. Pick fresh, healthy ingredients, and enjoy them with all of your senses!"
>
> – Sheri

Remember to let your kids help you wherever they can! Gathering the ingredients, measuring, cracking eggs, etc. You will see that we have food groups included with each recipe. Use this to open a healthy dialogue with your kids about what makes up the foods on their plate. (Ask them to figure out which food categories the Turkey Meatloaf and Mashed Potatoes are in, etc.) Try to have your older ones do the math to see if you would actually get a complete serving size out of each recipe. Yields are approximate – many will provide yummy leftovers!

Some of the recipes call for organic ingredients. Do you have to use only organic products? Will the recipes fail? No, the recipes will turn out, but there are several very good, sound reasons for choosing organic foods. Do some research with your kids about organic vs. conventionally grown foods. We strongly advocate that you support your local organic farmers. Read more about the local/organic movement online at www.localharvest.com.

## Which Came First? The Nutritionist or the Chef?

In the previous section, written by our nutritionist, Emily Harrison, we explained why each of the food categories are important. This section contains recipes by Sheri, who has been trained in making yummy, healthy foods. On the surface, some of the information might seem contradictory. Should you use heavy cream and butter when you cook? Well sometimes, sure, just not all the time, and be sure to control your portions!

We all believe that eating healthy should be simple. It is very important to teach your kids to eat real foods and to control the amount they eat. This means you have to educate yourself and your children about what healthy foods are and what healthy portion sizes are. If you have dietary restrictions, please make adjustments to the recipes provided.

## Some great substitutions:

- Instead of only using whole eggs (yolk and white), use ½ whole eggs and ½ egg whites.

- Substitute out cream, heavy cream, whipping cream, etc., in favor of skim or 1% milk.

- Use a smaller amount of butter than called for (especially if it is just being used as a "release" from the pan) or add a little canola or olive oil instead.

- Use non-stick cookware. It requires less oil/butter.

# Breakfast

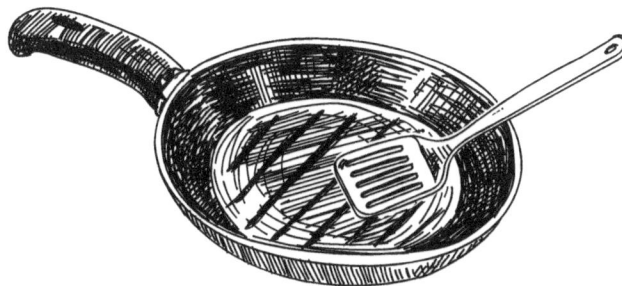

# Veggie Skillet *with* Potatoes & Eggs

**GRAINS** | **VEGGIES** | **DAIRY** | **PROTEIN**

*Prep Time: 15 minutes* | *Cook Time: 15 minutes* | *Yield: 6-8 servings*

2 Tablespoons canola oil (total – use 1 Tablespoon in each pan)

4 Yukon Gold potatoes, diced small

½ cup onion, diced small

½ cup fresh asparagus, sliced into ¼" rounds

½ cup grape tomatoes, cut in half

Salt and pepper

½ cup portabella mushrooms, sliced

8 eggs

Fresh herbs or cheese to top

**UTENSILS NEEDED:**
12" sauté pan, 10" sauté pan, whisk, rubber spatula, bowl

1. Add 1 Tablespoon of canola oil to each pan over high heat. In the large sauté pan, add potatoes and onions, and season with salt and pepper.

2. Cook until the potatoes are tender. Add the asparagus and grape tomatoes, season, and set aside.

3. In the second hot sauté pan, add the mushrooms. Season when they are cooked.

4. Add the eggs, season again, and cook to your liking (sunny side up, scrambled, fried).

5. Place the potatoes and veggies in the center of the plate, with the eggs and mushrooms on top. Top with fresh herbs or cheese.

Add your favorite cheese, veggies, meats, or meat alternatives, such as sundried tomatoes, jarred artichokes, spinach, sausages, ham, flavored tofu, shrimp, smoked salmon, or roasted garlic.

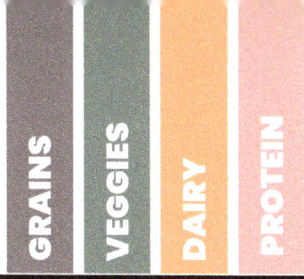

# Sweet Potato Hash *WITH* Eggs on English Muffins

GRAINS | VEGGIES | DAIRY | PROTEIN

*Prep Time: 15 minutes*   *Cook Time: 15 minutes*   *Yield: 4-6 servings*

1 Tablespoon canola oil

1 onion, diced small

4 sweet potatoes, peeled and diced small

Salt and pepper

½ pound favorite sausage, sliced to your liking (sundried tomato and basil tofurkey is really good)

1 red pepper, diced small

3 whole wheat English muffins

1 Tablespoon butter

6 eggs

**UTENSILS NEEDED:**
2–10" sauté pans, spatula, peeler, paring knife

1. Get sauté pan hot. Add oil, onions and potatoes, and season with salt and pepper.

2. Add sliced sausage and red pepper. Sauté everything until the potatoes are golden brown and the sausages are cooked.

3. Toast the English muffins and lightly butter. (You can alternatively use any favorite bread.)

4. In another sauté pan, add butter and crack the eggs in the pan to fry. Season the eggs with salt and pepper. When eggs are cooked to your liking, place on top of the sweet potato hash and serve over the muffins.

You can cook the eggs however you like: poached, scrambled, sunnyside up, etc. Use any potatoes too – Yukon Gold are yummy.

# Cinnamon Spiced Millet
## ~WITH~ Peaches & Craisins

*Prep Time: 5 minutes    Cook Time: 30 minutes (5 min. pressure cooker)    Yield: 4-6 servings*

1 cup millet (found in stores that sell bulk grains)

1 Tablespoon butter

½ teaspoon cinnamon

⅛ teaspoon ground cloves

1 pound frozen sliced peaches

4 cups mango nectar or apple juice (substitute water for some of the juice to reduce sugar)

½ teaspoon vanilla extract

½ cup craisins

**UTENSILS NEEDED:**
Measuring cup, sauté pan, fine strainer, 2-quart stainless steel saucepan (or pressure cooker), wooden spoon

1. Start by toasting the millet on medium-high heat in a sauté pan. When lightly golden brown, place in a fine strainer and rinse. Set aside. (This step makes it extra good.)

2. Place butter, cinnamon, cloves, and frozen peaches in the 2 quart saucepan or pressure cooker. Cook on medium-high until spices release their flavors (about 8 minutes). Add the toasted millet and stir.

3. Add juice and vanilla. Bring to a boil, then lower to a medium simmer (or put the top on the pressure cooker at this point).

4. Cook for approximately 30 minutes (5 minutes in a pressure cooker) or until the millet is done to your liking. Can be al dente (kinda firm) or very soft. There should be just enough liquid to make the millet creamy.

5. When done, fold in the craisins and serve with your homemade Turkey Sausage.

## MILLET IS A YUMMY GRAIN AND A NICE BREAK FROM OATMEAL!

- It cooks quicker in a pressure cooker, and you can adjust the "stock" you cook the millet in to go with the other flavors on your plate.

- Substitute apples and butternut squash for the peaches and craisins.

- Use leftovers for a side dish with dinner or to stuff a chicken!

- Try an Italian-inspired dish by pairing with sundried tomatoes, artichokes, and parmesan cheese.

- Great with pork, salmon, chicken, and lamb.

- You can add cheeses at the end – top with blue cheese, brie, or goat cheese.

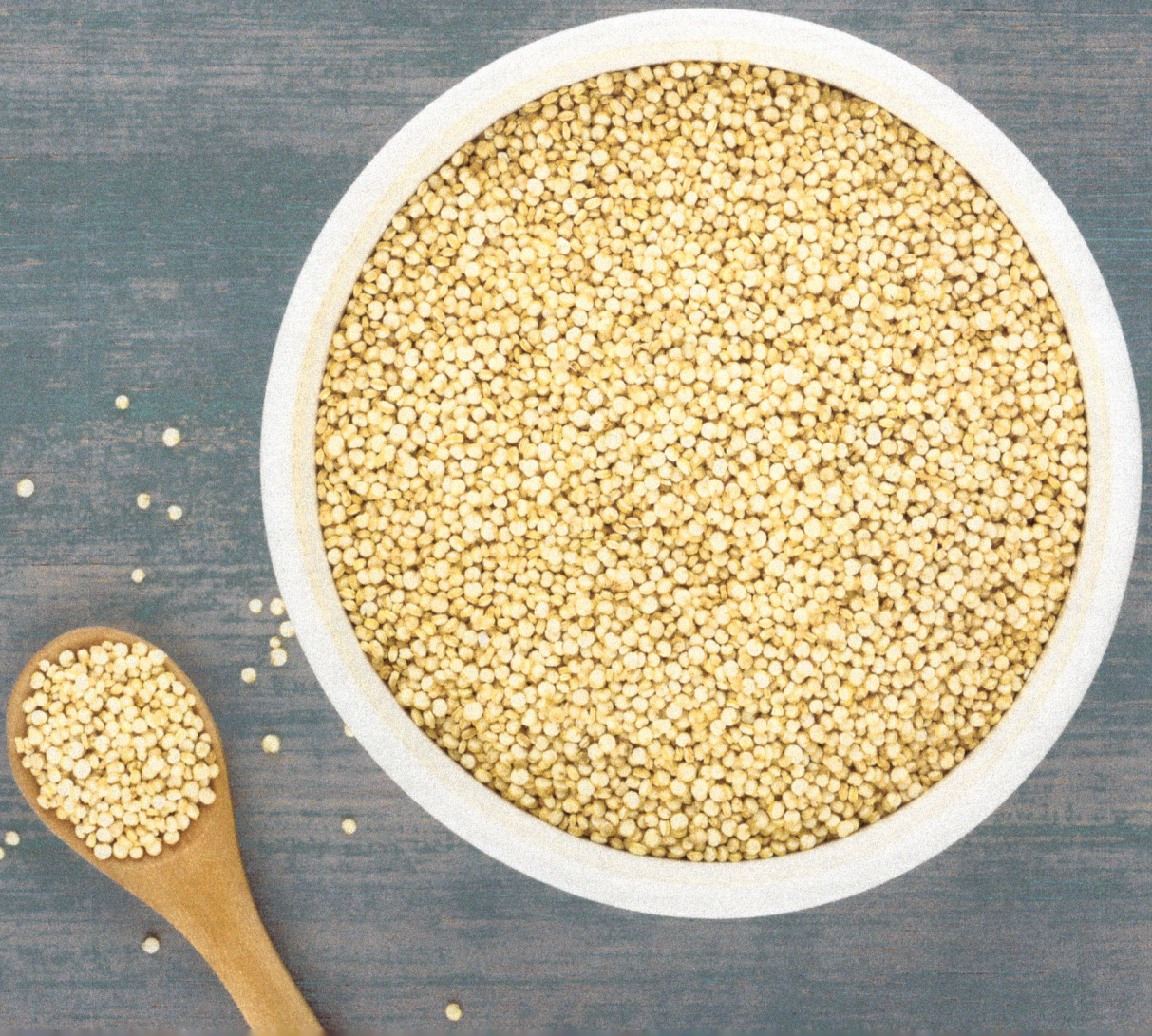

# Turkey Sausage

*Prep Time: 10 minutes* | *Cook Time: 15 minutes* | *Yield: 4-6 servings*

4 Tablespoons oil (canola or vegetable)

1 small onion, diced small

3 cloves of garlic, peeled and chopped

Salt and pepper to taste

½ red pepper, diced small

1 pound ground turkey

1 Tablespoon onion powder

½ teaspoon garlic powder

1 teaspoon ground fennel seed

½ teaspoon red pepper flakes (if your kids can handle it!)

**UTENSILS NEEDED:**
Two large sauté pans (one to cook onions and another to cook the sausage patties – if you use the same pan, it has to be nice and clean before you cook the patties), wooden spoon, spatula, bowl

1. Sauté onions and garlic with 1 Tablespoon of oil. Season with salt and freshly ground pepper. Cook until translucent. Add spices, and toast in the pan.

2. Add diced red pepper and season with salt and pepper. Remove from heat and place in a large bowl to cool.

3. When onion mix is cool, add turkey meat, onion powder, garlic powder, and ground fennel seeds. Mix well (your kids can do this with clean hands).

4. You can refrigerate at this point, then form the patties and cook in the morning.

5. Shape into patties, 2–3" across and ¼–½" thick. Try to keep thickness the same from edge to edge.

6. Heat oil in the sauté pan. Add patties and cook until golden brown and firm to the touch (about 8 minutes each side).

7. Serve with Sweet Potato Hash or whole wheat toast and fresh fruit.

### Why make your own sausage when you can just buy it at the store?

Processed meat products like sausage are packaged with many fillers and sulfites that your body doesn't need. It only takes a few minutes to make and freeze these! Make a double or triple batch and freeze for later.

# Vegetable Frittata ⟨WITH⟩ Whole Wheat Biscuit

| *Prep Time: 15 minutes* | *Cook Time: 25 minutes* | *Yield: 6-8 servings* |
|---|---|---|

2 Tablespoons butter

1 small onion, diced

1 cup mushrooms, sliced

½ cup grape tomatoes, cut in half

1 red pepper, diced

1 cup fresh spinach

Salt and pepper

8 eggs

¼ cup milk

¾ cup grated cheese (any variety your family likes)

Store-bought whole wheat biscuits, prepared

**UTENSILS NEEDED:**
Rubber spatula, 12" sauté pan (oven proof), 1 medium bowl, grater, whisk, wooden spoon

1. Preheat oven to 375°F.

2. Add butter to sauté pan over high heat.

3. Add onions, season with salt and pepper, and cook until translucent.

4. Add mushrooms, season, and cook until tender. Add tomatoes, red peppers, and spinach, then season. Turn heat down to low.

5. Crack eggs in a bowl, season with salt and pepper, and whisk in the milk.

6. Add egg mixture to the sauté pan, and move around with a wooden spoon. Top with grated cheese and put into the oven. Bake for about 15–20 minutes.

7. When eggs are thoroughly cooked, take out of the oven. You can use a rubber spatula to go around the edges of the frittata to release it. Put a plate on top of the sauté pan and flip it over onto the plate. Cut the frittata into wedges. Mind your portion sizes!

Serve with a whole wheat biscuit. Add any veggies and cheeses that your family prefers. My family especially likes this made with smoked salmon, bacon, diced breakfast sausage, etc.

Top pancakes with fresh sliced strawberries, blueberries, or diced cinnamon-spiced apples.

Use whatever bacon you like – turkey, beef, or veggie. Try nitrate-free bacon!

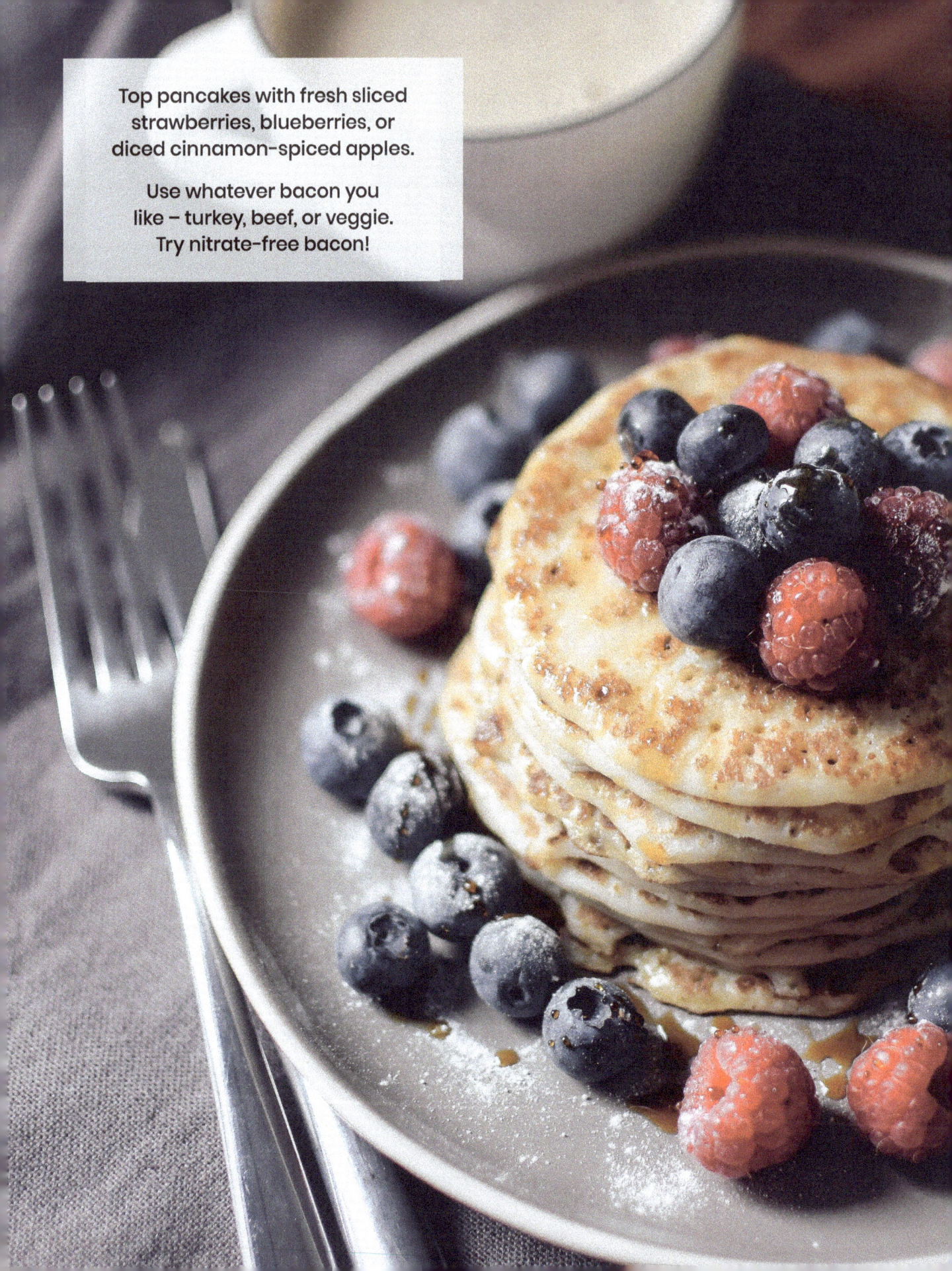

# Buttermilk Multigrain Pancakes ~WITH~ Berries & Bacon

GRAINS FRUITS PROTEIN EXTRAS

---

*Prep Time: 10 minutes*  |  *Cook Time: 20 minutes*  |  *Yield: 6-8 servings*

---

½ pound bacon, cooked to your liking

2 cups multigrain flour (mix whole wheat and white if you'd like)

2 teaspoons baking soda

2 teaspoons baking powder

½ teaspoon salt

5 Tablespoons organic sugar or agave nectar

1 teaspoon ground cinnamon

2 eggs

3 Tablespoons melted butter

2 ½–3 cups buttermilk

Canola oil for cooking

1 cup fresh blueberries

Maple syrup


**UTENSILS NEEDED:**
Griddle or large skillet, large bowl, medium bowl, whisk, metal spatula

1. Preheat the griddle or skillet.

2. Mix the flour, baking soda, baking powder, salt, sugar, and cinnamon in a large bowl. Mix with a whisk. (Using agave nectar? Mix in the next step).

3. In another bowl, whisk together the eggs, melted butter, and buttermilk. Add egg mixture to flour mixture, whisking until smooth.

4. Add some oil to the griddle, and pour in approximately 1–2 ounces of pancake batter.

5. Put several blueberries onto each pancake. (This keeps the blueberries from getting all mashed up into the batter and ensures everyone has an even number of blueberries – I hate that "who has more" argument in my house!)

6. When pancakes start to form small bubbles, flip over and cook on the other side. I like to add a little butter to the edges of the pancakes to crispen them up.

7. When cooked, place on a plate and top with some more fresh blueberries. Serve with bacon and syrup.

# French Toast ⟨with⟩ Fruit

GRAINS • FRUITS • PROTEIN • EXTRAS

*Prep Time: 10 minutes*   *Cook Time: 15 minutes*   *Yield: 4-6 servings*

6 eggs

¼ cup milk

⅛ teaspoon cinnamon

⅛ teaspoon vanilla

4–6 1" thick slices of ciabatta bread

3 Tablespoons canola oil

1 cup fresh or 8 ounces frozen berries

Butter

**UTENSILS NEEDED:**
Large bowl, spatula, whisk, griddle or large sauté pan, blender, small bowl, spoon

1. Start by heating the griddle or sauté pan on medium heat (around 300°F).

2. Crack eggs into large bowl, adding the milk, cinnamon, and vanilla. Whisk until blended.

3. Add ciabatta, turning on each side to let the bread soak up the egg mixture.

4. Put a little oil onto the griddle and add the soaked bread. Cook until golden brown, then flip to do the same on the other side. I like to add a little butter at the end to crisp the edges.

5. Place berries in a bowl to mix them up. Take ½ cup and blend in the blender. Add the blended berry juice to the mixed berries. Mix with a spoon and top the French toast with the berry mix.

Any favorite fruits or bread will work.

# Morning Snack

You want a morning snack to provide carbs, and the addition of dairy would be great as well. If your child is in school and they don't serve snack, make sure to pack something like a cheese stick or an apple in their lunch. Talk to your child's teacher about possibly incorporating a morning snack into the class routine.

Kids, especially those in school, need food to keep going. Make sure if they do get a snack at school, they are not being served candy or high-salt/high-fat chips.

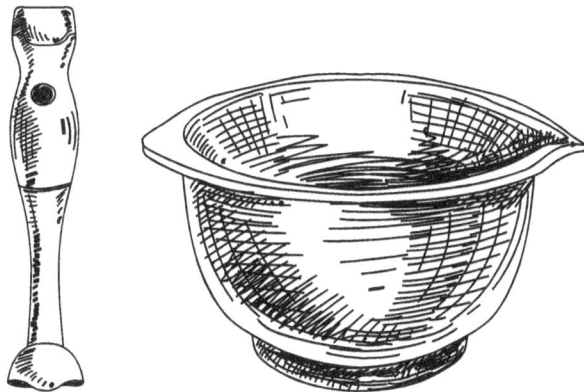

GRAINS　FRUITS　PROTEIN　EXTRAS

# Honey-Vanilla Granola

*Prep Time: 10 minutes*　　*Cook Time: 35 minutes*　　*Yield: 8-10 servings*

2 cups old-fashioned rolled oats

¼ cup each of:

- pecan pieces
- raisins
- halved cashews
- craisins
- diced small dates
- shelled sunflower seeds
- dried cherries
- diced dried mango
- pumpkin seeds
- small pretzels

1 Tablespoon ground cinnamon

1 Tablespoon vanilla extract

¼ cup organic brown sugar

¼ cup honey

¼ cup melted butter

½ Tablespoon salt

**UTENSILS NEEDED:**
Large bowl, 2 cookie sheets/trays, wooden spoon

1. Preheat oven to 300°F.

2. Toss everything in a large bowl.

3. Place on 2 sheet trays and bake 35 minutes, stirring occasionally.

4. Keep stored in airtight container.


**Great for breakfast too!**

You can use any favorite nuts and dried fruits. Great as a topping on yogurt, ice cream, cereal, or just as a snack.

FRUITS DAIRY PROTEIN

# Banana Fruit Smoothie

*Prep Time: 10 minutes*    *Cook Time: Zero*    *Yield: 2-4 servings*

1 cup skim milk (or ½ cup orange juice)

1 very ripe banana

1 teaspoon vanilla extract

½ cup peaches, fresh or frozen

½ cup strawberries, fresh or frozen

8 ounces vanilla yogurt

**UTENSILS NEEDED:**
Blender, rubber spatula

1.  Place all ingredients in the blender.

2.  Blend on medium until smooth.

Smoothies are the best quick breakfast food!

You can use any of your favorite fruits: mango, pitted cherries, blueberries, tropical mix, pineapple, etc.

GRAINS VEGGIES PROTEIN

# Lila G's Spinach Balls

*Prep Time: 10 minutes*     *Cook Time: 25-30 minutes*     *Yield: 10-12 balls*

10 ounces fresh spinach

4 slices of wheat bread

1 tablespoon Italian bread crumbs

½ pack firm tofu block

4 egg yolks

**UTENSILS NEEDED:**
Food processor, small bowl, large bowl, sheet pan

1. Put bread in food processor. When finely chopped, set aside in a small bowl.

2. Process spinach and put it into a large bowl.

3. Process tofu, egg yolks, and bread crumbs. Mix in with the spinach.

4. Form into balls, then roll in the chopped bread.

5. Spray a sheet pan and cook at 400°F for 25–30 minutes.

You can double this recipe, and it freezes well – just remove a few, heat, and serve when needed.

**GRAINS**  **VEGGIES**  **FRUITS**  **PROTEIN**

# Chicken & Apple Bites

*Prep Time: 10 minutes*          *Cook Time: 5-8 minutes*          *Yield: 20 bites*

1 apple, peeled, cored, and grated

2 skinless, boneless chicken breasts, cut into chunks

½ red onion, minced

1 tablespoon fresh parsley, minced

1 cup bread crumbs

1 tablespoon chicken stock or broth

Whole wheat flour

Peanut oil or olive oil

**UTENSILS NEEDED:**
Food processor, small bowl, skillet

1. Press out moisture in grated apple.

2. Process chicken, apple, onion, parsley, bread crumbs, and stock.

3. Roll into 20 balls. Roll in flour.

4. Place skillet over medium heat. Cook balls for 5–8 minutes (may take a little longer).

# More Snack Ideas

### Frozen grapes:

Place grapes into zipper bags or other closed container and put in the freezer overnight. Pull out when needed. Freezing concentrates the sugar in the grapes and makes them really yummy.

### Watermelon:

Place cubes of watermelon into zipper bags or other closed container. Put in the freezer overnight. Use them like ice cubes in fruit drinks or sparkling water.

### Cream cheese dips:

To a container of whipped cream cheese, add one or more of the following: pureed strawberries, pitted cherries, raspberries, mango slices, or pineapple. Whir briefly in a food processor, or mix in a bowl with a hand beater or stand mixer fitted with a paddle attachment.

### Vanilla yogurt with fruit:

Mix any whole or chopped fruits. Top with granola, or puree in the blender and add to the yogurt.

### Fruit kabobs of any flavor:

Large cubed fruits served on a skewer. Some fruits can be covered in crushed nuts, granola, chocolate, or sprinkles. Dip in yogurt then roll in covering. To make fresh freezy pops, place watermelon, grapes, cantaloupe, and pineapple skewers in the freezer.

# Lunch

One can hardly get away from mac-n-cheese. All kids seem to love it. If you must serve it five times a week, try to prepare its cousin, mac-n-peas, once in a while. Add some pretty green peas, give them some thinly sliced red peppers, and see who can connect the dots first! If you eat ham, there is some ready diced ham from the grocery store that you could also add.

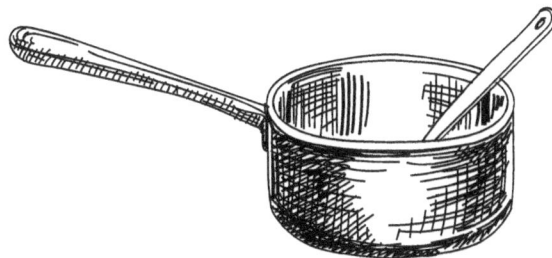

# Homemade Tomato Soup ⟨WITH⟩ Grilled Cheese

GRAINS · VEGGIES · DAIRY · PROTEIN · EXTRAS

*Prep Time: 20 minutes    Cook Time: 1 hour & 35 minutes    Yield: 4-6 servings*

4 Tablespoons olive oil

3 medium onions, diced small

8 garlic cloves, peeled

3 29-ounce cans of tomatoes, diced or whole peeled (flavored if you like) OR 10 cups fresh tomatoes, diced

3 bay leaves

Salt and pepper

8 slices whole wheat bread (or your favorite type – cut into shapes to control portions)

8 thick slices of mild cheddar cheese

2 Tablespoons softened butter

**UTENSILS NEEDED:**
3-quart, heavy bottomed stainless steel soup pot or saucepan, wooden spoon, 10" sauté pan

1. In a heavy-bottomed saucepan, add olive oil, bay leaves, onions, and garlic. Sauté on medium heat, and season with salt and black pepper. Cook until tender.

2. Add tomatoes. Stir around, seasoning with salt and pepper. Cook until great flavor develops (this can take anywhere from a half hour to an hour).

3. Add fresh basil if you'd like. Put through a food mill or blend in a blender for a couple of seconds – too much and it will turn pink. You can also put the soup through a strainer to get all the seeds out – just push it through with a ladle.

4. Taste for seasoning and adjust as needed.

5. For the sandwiches, start by heating a sauté pan.

6. Lightly butter the outside of each slice of bread and place in the sauté pan.

7. Add one slice of cheese, then the other piece of bread on top with the butter side up.

8. Cook until golden brown on each side, making sure the cheese has melted nicely. Let the sandwiches rest for a couple of minutes.

9. Ladle the soup into bowls, and cut the sandwiches in halves or quarters.

10. Serve it up!

Leftover tomato soup can be used for pasta or pizza sauce (use very lightly). Using this soup as a base, you can add all kinds of wonderful things like fennel, carrots, roasted red peppers, or corn.

Cheese sandwiches can consist of your favorite cheese: seasoned fresh mozzarella with basil, smoked gouda, goat cheese seasoned with basil and fresh black pepper, brie, gorgonzola, etc.

# Veggie Pasta ⟨WITH⟩ Marinara
## *(leftover Tomato Soup)*

| *Prep Time: 15 minutes* | *Cook Time: 20 minutes* | *Yield: 4-6 servings* |
|---|---|---|

½ pound pasta (spaghetti, vermicelli, penne, etc.)

1 cup mushrooms, sliced

½ cup carrots, sliced and quartered

½ cup zucchini, sliced and quartered

½ cup yellow squash, sliced and quartered

½ pound fresh spinach

2 cups leftover tomato soup

2 Tablespoons olive oil

¼ cup parmesan cheese, freshly grated

Salt and pepper

**UTENSILS NEEDED:**
3 quart saucepan, 2 quart saucepan, wooden spoon, grater

1. Bring salted water to a boil for the pasta. Cook pasta to your liking.

2. Heat a large saucepan until very hot, then add olive oil. Sauté mushrooms and season with salt and pepper.

3. Add the carrots, zucchini, and yellow squash. Season. Sauté until tender.

4. Add tomato soup. Bring up to a boil, then reduce heat to a simmer.

5. Add drained pasta to the veggie and tomato sauce. Add spinach, then toss.

6. Grate fresh parmesan over the top and serve.

Use whole wheat pasta and leftover veggies from the night before.

# Honey Baked Chicken Fingers

**GRAINS  PROTEIN  EXTRAS**

*Prep Time: 15 minutes*    *Cook Time: 20-25 Minutes*    *Yield: 4-6 servings*

2 eggs

2 Tablespoons honey

1 teaspoon granulated garlic

2 teaspoons extra virgin olive oil

2 cups panko bread crumbs (or cornflake crumbs, or bread crumbs)

1½ pounds chicken tenders, cut into 2" pieces (make sure all pieces are the same size)

5 Tablespoons oil (canola or vegetable)

Salt and pepper

**UTENSILS NEEDED:**
2 medium bowls, ½ sheet tray or cookie sheet, tongs, whisk

1. Preheat oven to 425°F. Coat sheet tray/cookie sheet with the oil.

2. Whisk eggs with honey in a large bowl. In another bowl, place panko and season with garlic, salt, and extra virgin olive oil.

3. Season chicken pieces with salt and pepper. Dredge the chicken in the honey/egg mixture, then dredge in the bowl of seasoned panko. (Use one hand for the wet mixture and one for the dry mixture to avoid battering your own fingers!)

4. Place on a cookie sheet, not touching each other. Bake for about 20 minutes, or until the nuggets are golden brown. At the 10 minute mark, you may want to check them and turn them over to ensure both sides are browning.

5. Cut one in half to make sure they are cooked through. Serve with steamed green beans and a nice, fresh salad to get your veggies in!

Flavors can be added to the egg whites with different sauces: BBQ, Buffalo, mustard, hoisen, etc. You can also add wheat germ to the breadcrumbs for extra fiber.

Bread and bake a double batch, then freeze the extra. To use, just heat up in the oven.

# Black Beans & Rice

*Prep Time: 20 minutes*     *Cook Time: 1-2 hours*     *Yield: 10-12 servings*

2 small onions, diced (1–2 cups)

3 cloves garlic, chopped

2 Tablespoons extra virgin olive oil

3 carrots, diced (1–2 cups)

1 cup celery, diced

15 ounces canned diced tomatoes (can be flavored – Italian, Mexican, etc.) **Do not drain; the juice will add flavor.**

2 Tablespoons cumin

Salt for flavor

1 pound black beans

Water

3 bay leaves

**UTENSILS NEEDED:**
3-quart saucepan, wooden spoon

## BLACK BEANS

1.  Start by sautéing the onions with the garlic in a little extra virgin olive oil.

2.  Add the carrots and celery. Season with salt. Add the tomatoes and cumin. Stir around to toast the cumin and release the flavor of the tomatoes.

3.  Add dried beans and bay leaves.

4.  Add water to cover beans by 3 inches. Bring to a boil, then bring down to a simmer. Cook uncovered until the beans are tender (about 1 ½ to 2 hours).

Don't soak the beans. Not only do they not need it, but the process of overnight soaking reduces the beany wonderfulness of this most basic of human foodstuffs.

Cooked beans freeze really well, so you can make a huge batch and freeze in serving sizes, so you'll always have homemade beans on hand. If you are in a rush, use canned beans instead.

3 cups long grain rice
(jasmine, basmati,
or white)

4 ½ cups water

1 Tablespoon salt

**UTENSILS NEEDED:**
2-quart saucepan with lid,
fork to fluff the rice

## RICE

1. The basic ratio for cooking rice is 1–1 ½ cups of water to 1 cup of rice.

2. Place rice, water, and salt into a 2-quart saucepan – either on the stove top covered at medium heat, or in the oven covered at 350°F for 30 minutes. If you have a pressure cooker, follow your manufacturer's instructions for the length of cooking time and optimal pressure.

### Options for Rice:
Add kaffir lime leaves to the pot while cooking for an Asian flavor (remove before serving).

Add bay leaves, diced carrots, zucchini, peas, and/or asparagus. You can use chicken, beef, or vegetable stock instead of water for extra flavor. If you are adding tomatoes or another juicy item, reduce the amount of water used. Try with brown rice for a yummy, healthy alternative!

### Options for Black Beans:
Add to Quinoa Salad with cooked fresh corn, lime, and cilantro. Have the leftovers for Fajita Night, quesadillas, or nachos.

# Marinated Noodles ⊰WITH⊱ Veggies & Peanut Sauce

GRAINS  VEGGIES  PROTEIN  EXTRAS

---

*Prep Time: 20 minutes*     *Cook Time: 15 Minutes*     *Yield: 6-8 servings*

---

1 pound fresh lo mein noodles (you can substitute whole wheat spaghetti, kumat, soba, or any thick noodle)

3 Tablespoons sesame oil

3 Tablespoons sweet soy sauce (it's thicker than regular soy sauce and has less salt)

2 Tablespoons balsamic vinegar

1 Tablespoon sweet chili sauce (I like Mae Ploy brand)

Salt to flavor the pasta water

½ cup shredded carrots

½ cup blanched broccoli

½ cup cooked edamame beans

½ cup red pepper, julienned

**UTENSILS NEEDED:**
3-quart saucepan, whisk, 1 large bowl, 2 small bowls, tongs

## NOODLES

1.  In a small bowl combine sesame oil, sweet soy sauce, balsamic vinegar, and sweet chili sauce. Whisk together. Have ready to put over hot pasta.

2.  Bring water to boil in the pot. Add salt for flavor. Cook pasta until done to your liking. Drain.

3.  Place drained pasta in a large bowl and add dressing while still hot (the pasta will absorb the dressing).

4.  Add veggies. Can serve immediately or refrigerate and serve cold.

ABC Brand is my favorite for sweet soy sauce. It's available at Asian markets or by mail order.

¾ cup peanut butter (smooth or chunky)

4 Tablespoons sweet soy sauce (can substitute regular)

2 Tablespoons ginger, peeled and microplaned or finely grated or jarred crushed ginger

¾ cup coconut milk

Warm water to thin

## PEANUT SAUCE

1. Whisk everything together in a bowl until smooth. Add warm water to thin the peanut dressing to your liking.

2. Drizzle over marinated pasta and veggies.

Keep some of the lo mein separate for the kids in case they don't want to eat peanut sauce.

Great with grilled salmon, shrimp, chicken of any sort, flavored tofu, sliced flank steak, and any style pork.

Sauté your favorite veggies: sliced shiitake or portobello mushrooms, eggplant, or chopped baby bok choy, and then top with fresh bean sprouts or julienned Napa cabbage. You can always omit the peanut sauce.

GRAINS VEGGIES PROTEIN

# Chicken Noodle Soup

*Prep Time: 20 minutes*  | *Cook Time: 45 Minutes* | *Yield: 6-8 servings*

1 chicken carcass (from last night's chicken dinner!)

3 carrots, diced small

3 stalks celery, diced small

1 large onion, peeled and diced small

8 cloves garlic, peeled and sliced

3 bay leaves

Salt and pepper

Pasta (whatever is in the cupboard)

**UTENSILS NEEDED:**
3-quart saucepan,
1 medium bowl

1. Place the carcass in a pot and cover with cold water (approximately 2 quarts).

2. Season all veggies with salt and pepper. Add to the chicken pot with bay leaves. Bring to a boil, then reduce to a simmer. Cook until it has a great flavor (approximately 40 minutes).

3. While chicken stock is cooking, cook pasta to your liking. Cook, drain, and cool.

4. Reserving the liquid and veggies, strain chicken mixture. Discard the carcass. Add veggies back into stock.

5. If you have any chicken left from the night before, chop it up into bite-sized pieces and add to soup. Add noodles and serve!

Add fresh herbs like basil, cilantro, or oregano. Substitute tomatoes for some of the water.

Add peeled/chopped ginger and chopped lemongrass, and serve with Asian vegetables and rice noodles or rice.

For Mexican style, add tomatoes, corn, rice, cilantro, and a squeeze of fresh lime. Try with white beans instead of pasta.

Never known what to do with a parsnip? Put some in chicken soup!

# Afternoon Snack

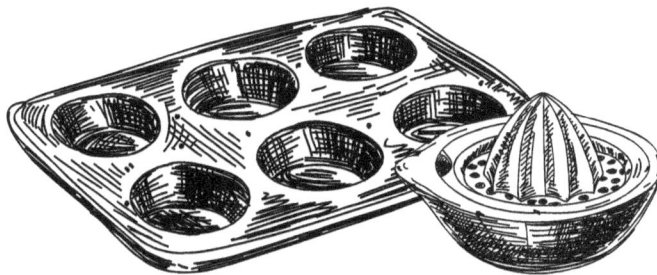

# Hummus ⟨WITH⟩ Whole Wheat Pita

GRAINS VEGGIES PROTEIN

*Prep Time: 20 minutes*  |  *Cook Time: Zero*  |  *Yield: 10-12 servings*

30 ounces canned garbanzo beans/chickpeas, drained

2 Tablespoons tahini paste (a sesame seed product)

3 Tablespoons roasted garlic cloves, peeled (OR 1 Tablespoon roasted granulated garlic)

2 Tablespoons cumin, ground

Salt

White pepper

3 Tablespoons lemon juice (one large lemon)

Whole wheat pita to make chips

Butter

**UTENSILS NEEDED:**
Food processor fitted with metal blade (or blender), rubber spatula

1. In food processor or blender, add drained garbanzo beans, Tahini, roasted garlic, cumin, salt, and freshly ground white pepper.

2. Blend and puree until smooth, stopping and scraping the bowl with a rubber spatula several times.

3. Add lemon juice when smooth. Don't add lemon juice too soon – you'll have chunky hummus.

4. Serve with pita chips and veggies.

I like to sauté my pita bread on both sides in a small amount of butter to crispen it up a little.

Hummus makes a great spread for sandwiches, whole wheat tortillas, and flatbreads of all flavors. Combine with black olives, sprouts, lettuce, tomatoes, roasted tomatoes, or thinly sliced cucumbers.

Great for packing a lunch!

# Flatbread ⧼WITH⧽ Caramelized
# Onions, Red Peppers, & Goat Cheese

**GRAINS VEGGIES DAIRY EXTRAS**

*Prep Time: 20 minutes* | *Cook Time: 20 minutes* | *Yield: 6-8 servings*

4 flatbreads, any flavor, or Sardinian flatbread (found at Italian grocer or farmers' markets)

3 sprigs of thyme, lightly chopped

2 red peppers, roasted and julienned

4 ounces crumbled goat cheese (or any favorite cheese – I love gorgonzola!)

3 onions, julienned

Salt and pepper

1 teaspoon extra virgin olive oil

**UTENSILS NEEDED:**
Cookie sheet, sauté pan, wooden spoon, metal spatula

1. Preheat oven 400°F. Start by cooking the onions with extra virgin olive oil in a sauté pan. Season with salt and pepper. Cook until tender and golden brown.

2. Add fresh thyme to the onions. Cool down on a plate.

3. Place the flatbread onto cookie sheets, 2 per tray.

4. Evenly spread the caramelized onions and julienned roasted red pepper on the flatbreads.

5. Drizzle a little extra virgin olive oil onto each flatbread. Sprinkle with a little sea salt and fresh ground pepper.

6. Top with the crumbled goat cheese, and bake until golden brown or cheese is just melted.

7. Plate and serve.

There are many flavors you can add – just don't add too much, or they won't get crispy.

GRAINS | VEGGIES | DAIRY | PROTEIN | EXTRAS

# Corn Muffins

*Prep Time: 20 minutes*  *Cook Time: 25 minutes*  *Yield: 10-12 servings*

1 ¼ cup all-natural stone ground cornmeal

1 cup organic all-purpose flour

½ cup organic sugar

¼ teaspoon salt

1 teaspoon baking soda

2 teaspoons baking powder

3 eggs

¼ cup melted salted butter (½ stick)

1 cup milk or buttermilk

½ cup cheddar cheese, grated

1 cup corn, cooked or frozen

2 Tablespoons granulated organic sugar

**UTENSILS NEEDED:**
Muffin tin, stand mixer with whisk attachment or hand beater, measuring spoons, grater

1. Preheat oven to 425°F.

2. Butter and sugar muffin tins (use regular size – not jumbo!).

3. In a stand mixer or a large bowl, add all dry ingredients (except final 2 Tablespoons of sugar). Whisk around until blended.

4. Add eggs and melted butter. Slowly add the milk.

5. Add the cheese and corn. Mix all ingredients until well blended.

6. Fill muffin tins with the corn batter until ¾ full. Sprinkle a little sugar on the top of each muffin.

7. Bake for about 20–25 minutes or until a toothpick inserted in the middle comes out clean.

8. Let rest for 15 minutes before serving.

Leftover muffins make great stuffing.

# Mango Salsa ⌐WITH⌐ Chips & Veggies

**GRAINS** **VEGGIES** **FRUITS** **DAIRY**

*Prep Time: 20 minutes*   *Cook Time: Zero*   *Yield: 4-6 servings*

2 ripe mangos, peeled and diced small

1 carrot, peeled and diced small

1 cucumber, peeled and diced small

1 Asian pear, peeled and diced small

1 lime, juiced

1 cup orange juice

Fresh mint and basil, julienned

Salt and pepper to taste

**UTENSILS NEEDED:**
Bowl, chef's knife, spoon, peeler

1. Add fruits and veggies into a bowl and season with salt and pepper.

2. Add juices and mix with a spoon.

3. Add chopped fresh mint and basil.

4. Serve with any favorite chips: tortilla, pita, etc.

**Also good with cut-up celery, broccoli, and cauliflower.**

Popcorn will be freshest within the first four hours, but I've eaten it up to a day later and it was great.

You'll have extra rosemary oil (about 4 ¼ cups) left over. Place in the fridge or covered on the counter, and it will last three weeks – longer if it's in the fridge. You can use the oil for marinades, pasta sauces, salad dressings, and sautés.

Add fresh parmesan cheese to the popcorn as it comes out from popping. Try different salts, roasted granulated garlic, garlic salt, smoked salt, etc.

Make your own flavored salts. Just finely zest a lemon, lime, or orange – let it dry out on a sheet tray, sitting in the oven overnight. On the next day, mix it with some sea salt. You can keep the flavors individual or create your own custom mixes.

You can do the same thing to create flavored sugars. Add craisins, raisins, nuts, etc. Make a signature flavor for your family!

# Rosemary Popcorn

*Prep Time: 30 mins to prepare oil   Cook Time: 10 minutes   Yield: 10-12 servings*

5 ounces fresh rosemary

2 Tablespoons kosher salt

5 cups oil blend (3 ½ cups canola to 1 ½ cups extra virgin olive oil)

Additional ½ ounce rosemary springs (2–3)

1 ½ cups organic yellow popcorn

⅔ to ¾ cups rosemary oil (about 4–6 ounces)

Fine sea salt

**UTENSILS NEEDED:**
1- to 3-quart sauce pot with lid, 1- to 2-quart sauce pot, 1 very large bowl, tongs

## ROSEMARY OIL (YOU WILL HAVE LEFTOVER)

1. Place oil in a 2 quart pot on medium heat, and add 4 ounces of fresh rosemary, breaking the stems into the oil to release the flavors.

2. Add salt and bring to a boil.

3. Remove from heat and set aside.

## POPPING THE POPCORN

4. Place popcorn in a 3-quart saucepan. Add just enough rosemary oil to cover the popcorn, but not so much that the kernels are swimming.

5. Add 2 sprigs of fresh rosemary, put the lid on, and turn to high heat to get good steam action. Popcorn will start popping vigorously. Keep the lid on and shake the pot back and forth over the heat. Have a large bowl, a big spoon, and sea salt ready.

6. When popping starts to slow down, carefully remove the lid, take some of the popped corn out with your spoon, and put it into the large bowl. Sprinkle with a little sea salt.

7. Allow remainder of corn to finish popping, then turn off the heat. Add the rest of the popcorn to the bowl, season with salt, and toss the popcorn around. Add more fresh rosemary to garnish.

# More Snack Ideas

Make different spreads for sandwiches or wraps:

- Combine seasoned avocado with light sour cream or cream cheese, chopped cilantro, hint of lime, and tomatoes.

- Puree leftover cooked beans and add flavorings or sour cream. Spread on tortillas or pitas, or serve with crackers as a dip.

- Add veggies over hummus spread: sprouts, tomato, chopped lettuce, cucumber slices, shaved carrots, black olive slices, roasted peppers, or cooked or jarred artichokes.

The list goes on...

# Dinner

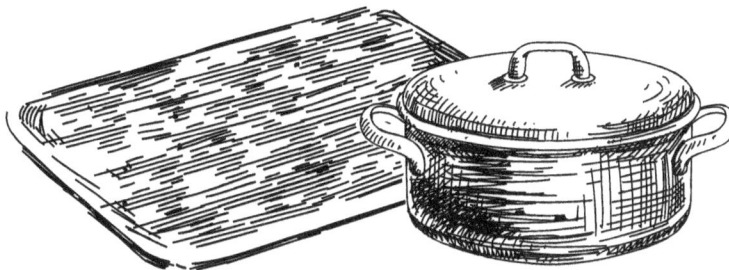

# Roasted Pork Loin ⟨with⟩ Black Bean & Corn Quinoa

**GRAINS · VEGGIES · PROTEIN**

*Prep Time: 15 minutes*   *Cook Time: 1 ½ hours*   *Yield: 4-6 servings*

Pork loin (about 3 pounds)

3 Tablespoons extra virgin olive oil

3 cups quinoa

3 bay leaves

1 onion, diced

6 garlic cloves, peeled and sliced

2 cans seasoned black beans

2 cups cooked yellow corn

1 cup grape tomatoes, halved

3 Tablespoons cilantro or flat Italian parsley, chopped

1 Tablespoon ground cumin

2 limes, juiced

Salt and pepper

**UTENSILS NEEDED:**
Sheet tray or cookie sheet, wire rack, sauce pan, wooden spoon

1. Preheat oven to 375°F.

2. Cut pork loin in half or into thirds. Season the top, bottom, and all sides with salt and pepper. Place on a wire rack on a ½ sheet tray or cookie sheet with sides.

3. Place in the oven on the top shelf. Approximate cooking time should be an hour (depending on the loin size and your particular oven).

4. Spread the quinoa on another sheet pan and put into the oven to toast until golden brown, about 3–5 minutes. Toasting before cooking brings out a wonderful nutty flavor.

5. While the pork is cooking, in a 4-quart saucepan, place extra virgin olive oil, onions, and garlic. Sauté on medium heat. Season with salt and pepper, and add bay leaves.

6. When onions are translucent, add cumin and approximately 3 quarts of water. Bring to a boil, taste for flavor, and adjust seasonings to your preference.

7. Add toasted quinoa and cook until the grain looks translucent (about 12 minutes). Drain out liquid, add seasoned black beans, corn, and tomatoes, and toss. Add lime juice and parsley.

8. Remove pork from the oven. Allow to rest for a few minutes, then slice or fillet to serve.

**Leftovers make great lunches!**

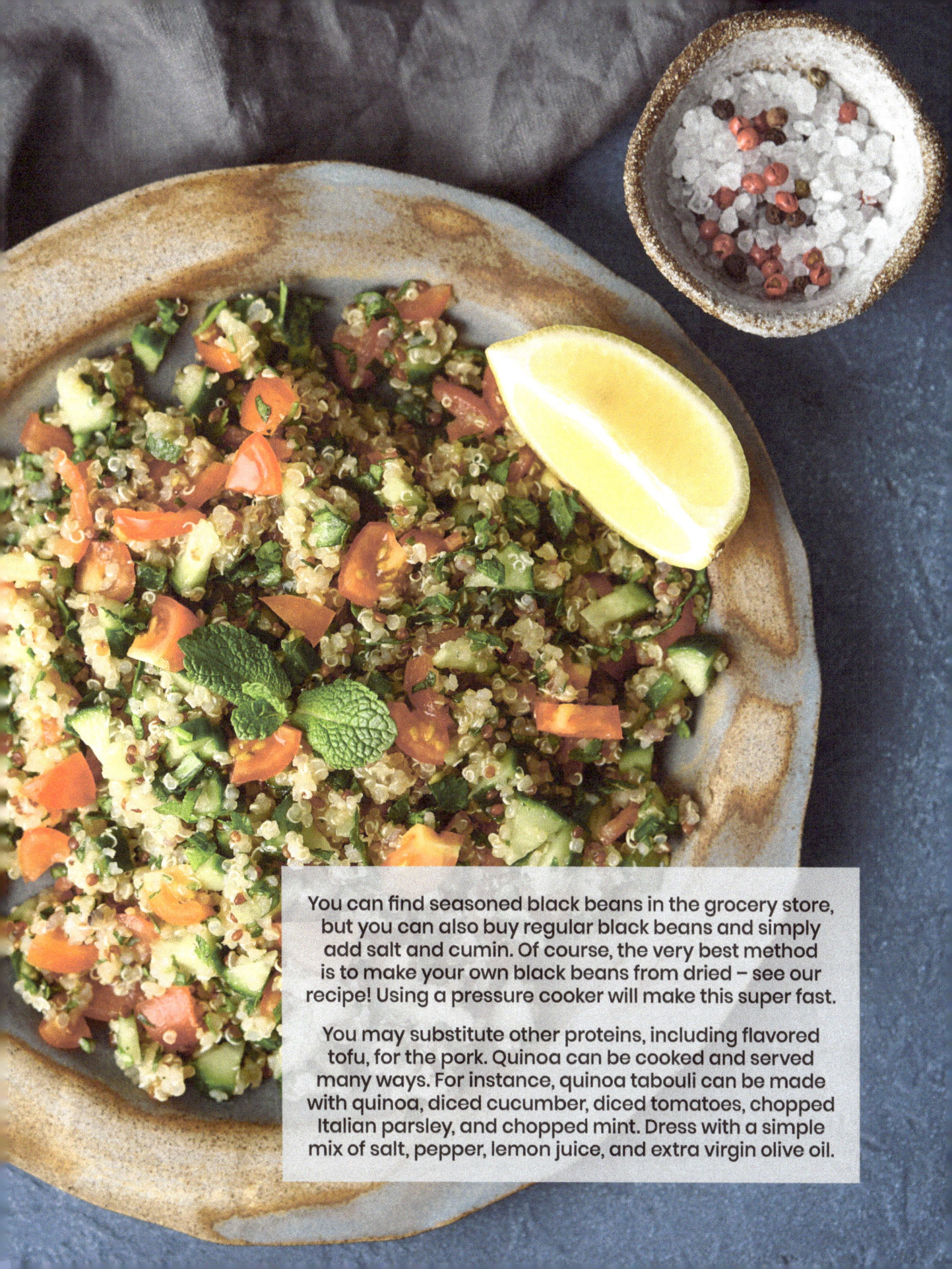

You can find seasoned black beans in the grocery store, but you can also buy regular black beans and simply add salt and cumin. Of course, the very best method is to make your own black beans from dried – see our recipe! Using a pressure cooker will make this super fast.

You may substitute other proteins, including flavored tofu, for the pork. Quinoa can be cooked and served many ways. For instance, quinoa tabouli can be made with quinoa, diced cucumber, diced tomatoes, chopped Italian parsley, and chopped mint. Dress with a simple mix of salt, pepper, lemon juice, and extra virgin olive oil.

# Grilled Salmon ⟨with⟩ Corn Succotash

**GRAINS** **VEGGIES** **DAIRY** **PROTEIN**

*Prep Time: 15 minutes*     *Cook Time: 15 minutes*     *Yield: 4-6 servings*

4 fresh salmon fillets
(5 ounces each)

2 cups corn, fresh or frozen

½ cup lima beans, fresh
or frozen

½ cup edamame beans,
fresh or frozen

1 red pepper, diced

½ cup green beans, fresh
or frozen

1 medium onion, diced

2 cloves garlic, chopped

½ cup grape tomatoes,
halved

1 Tablespoon butter

1 Tablespoon olive oil

Salt and pepper

Whole wheat dinner rolls

**UTENSILS NEEDED:**
Outdoor grill or grill pan,
tongs, sauté pan, wooden
spoon

1. Drizzle each filet with olive oil and season on both sides with freshly ground white pepper and salt.

2. In the sauté pan, over medium heat, add butter, garlic, and onion. Season with salt and pepper.

3. When cooked through, add corn, red pepper, and all the beans. Season.

4. Toss the vegetables or move them with the wooden spoon to ensure even cooking. Bring to a boil and cook for just a few minutes, or until everything is warmed up.

5. Add the grape tomatoes and cook until tomatoes are at your desired consistency (some people like them al dente and some prefer tomatoes very soft).

6. Start up the grill or heat the grill pan on the stove top until smoky. Be sure to have your vent hood on if you are using a grill pan.

When the grill is hot, use a grill brush on it, and then wipe down with a little oil on a towel before you begin cooking. Use care, of course. This will help to release the salmon.

7. When grill is very hot, add the salmon on a diagonal (with the presentation side down first). Cook for three minutes. Rotate salmon diagonally and cook for another three minutes (this will give you those lovely diamond shaped grill marks).

   The salmon should release from the pan easily; if not, cook until it releases. Do not try to force it if it's not ready. Turn salmon onto the other side and cook for another three minutes, rotating again.

8. Serve the salmon with succotash and rolls.

Instead of salmon, use grilled pork chops, pork loin, lamb chops, lamb loin, or flavored tofu. You can also add fresh julienned basil, chives, or Italian parsley for extra flavor.

# Roast Chicken *with* Potatoes & Carrots

| *Prep Time: 12 minutes* | *Cook Time: 1 ½ hours* | *Yield: 4-6 servings* |
|---|---|---|

1 large whole chicken (about 3 ½ pounds)

4 large Yukon Gold potatoes

4 large carrots

2 medium yellow onions, peeled

6 cloves of garlic, peeled

2 bay leaves

Salt and white pepper

**UTENSILS NEEDED:**
Roasting pan or casserole dish, tongs, chef's knife

1. Preheat oven to 375°F.

2. No need to peel veggies, just wash and cut into one-inch cubes.

3. Place veggies into a roasting pan or casserole dish. Add garlic, bay leaves, and season with salt and freshly ground white pepper.

4. Season chicken with salt and freshly ground pepper inside and out, then place on top of the veggies.

5. Place into oven. Cook approximately 1 hour – check if chicken is golden brown in color. If drumstick moves easily, chicken is done.

6. Remove chicken from oven. Allow to rest for a few minutes. Remove chicken to cutting board. Slice chicken into serving sizes and serve with veggies.

Use organic free-range chicken if it's available. It simply tastes better.

Once you've taken all the meat off the bone, make a quick chicken stock while you are eating dinner.

Just throw the carcass in a stockpot, add some carrots, celery, whole peeled garlic cloves, salt and pepper. Cover with water, bring to a boil, then turn down to a low simmer. Let cool and save in the fridge for chicken soup the next day!

You can use the same recipe and substitute a pot roast, but cook for about 2 hours.

# Asian Stir Fry

*Prep Time: 15 minutes*    *Cook Time: 15 minutes*    *Yield: 6-8 servings*

2 cups cooked rice (left over from black beans and rice)

1 pound protein of your choice, already cooked (Use up leftovers!)

1 cup peas, fresh or frozen

1 cup baby carrots, peeled or carrots cut into small pieces

1 cup broccoli florets

1 cup bean sprouts

2 Tablespoon soy sauce (to your liking)

1 Tablespoon fresh ginger, minced

1 Tablespoon garlic, peeled and sliced (3–4 cloves)

1 Tablespoon canola oil (or peanut oil, which can also withstand very high heat)

**UTENSILS NEEDED:**
Wok (or heavy sauté pan), wooden spoon, fry pan

1. Start by getting the wok or heavy sauté pan hot.

2. Add the oil, toss in the ginger and garlic, and then season with salt. Move it around.

3. Bring the heat down to medium. Add the carrots, toss, and season again.

4. Add the peas and broccoli, toss and season.

5. Add the rice (or you can heat it in the microwave if you'd like it plain).

6. Add soy sauce and toss.

7. Add your meat, fish, or tofu. Turn to heat evenly.

8. Serve sprinkled with bean sprouts.

If you have any leftover veggies, meat, or fish to use up, just julienne and add to heat through.

# Thin Pizza Dough

*Prep Time: one hour*     *Cook Time: 20 minutes*     *Yield: 6-8 servings*

⅓ cup warm water (about 112°F, to activate yeast)

½ package dry yeast

1 ⅓ cups flour (mix whole wheat and plain if you'd like)

1 egg

½ teaspoon salt

1 teaspoon extra virgin olive oil

Extra flour for kneading

**UTENSILS NEEDED:**
rolling pin, ½ sheet tray or cookie sheet (see note on kitchen equipment), stand mixer with paddle, sauté pan

If you don't have a big mixer, you can add ingredients by hand and knead it yourself to build muscles, or head to a friend's house to make dough together.

1. Place warm water and yeast in a stand mixer bowl. Let activate for a minute.

2. Add the rest of the ingredients.

3. Using the paddle attachment, move the dough at low to medium speed until it all comes together, forming a ball. (Or get busy with your hands. Push away, fold over, ½ turn, repeat.)

4. Cover the dough with plastic wrap and leave it in a warm spot for about an hour, until it doubles in size.

5. Punch the dough down, then put it on a floured surface. Dust the top with a light cover of flour. Roll out into one ⅛ inch thick large or several small rounds (yields 8–10 individual 6-inch pizzas).

6. For individual pizzas, cook in a sauté pan with a little olive oil for three minutes on each side. For a single large pizza, roll out the dough to fit onto a ½ sheet pan. Bake at 375°F for 20 minutes.

You can double or triple this recipe, roll out, cook, and freeze to have handy, or simply freeze the raw dough balls by wrapping tightly in plastic wrap and enclosing in a zip lock. They should last for at least a month when frozen. Take them out in the morning, and they'll be ready for dinner.

# Thin Pizza Toppings

*Prep Time: 10 minutes*   *Cook Time: 20 minutes*   *Yield: 6-8 servings*

29 ounces canned diced tomatoes with Italian seasoning

½ small can tomato paste

1 ½ cups grated mozzarella cheese

Salt and pepper

**UTENSILS NEEDED:**
Sauté pan, wooden spoon, grater, ½ sheet tray or cookie sheet

1. Preheat oven to 450°F. In a sauce pan, add the tomatoes and tomato paste, and season with salt and pepper. You can also season with garlic salt if your kids like garlic.

2. Cook on medium heat until the liquid has evaporated and the sauce is thick (about 10 minutes).

3. Spray or, with a paper towel, rub a thin layer of oil onto the ½ sheet tray (this will yield a crispier crust). Place your pre-cooked pizza dough on the tray; 2–3 small pizza rounds should fit.

4. Top pizza dough with tomato sauce and mozzarella. Add other toppings, being careful to not get them too heavy.

5. Bake until cheese is melted and crust is crispy, about 8–10 minutes.

This is a good way to add veggies to a fun meal. If your kids are cheese pizza eaters, serve a side salad or steamed veggies. The message is that while veggies are not optional, the way you eat them is.

It's easy to make your own pizza sauce, and it won't have the high fructose corn syrup or other additives the store bought kind does. Pre-shredded cheese is also sometimes full of additives. Most school-aged kids can learn to grate cheese.

GRAINS VEGGIES PROTEIN EXTRAS

# Turkey Meatloaf

*Prep Time: 15 minutes*    *Cook Time: 35 Minutes*    *Yield: 6-8 servings*

3 pounds ground turkey

6 Tablespoons Worcestershire sauce

1 large onion, diced small

5 cloves garlic, peeled and chopped

2 carrots, diced small

2 eggs

25 saltine or Club crackers, crushed

2 Tablespoons canola oil

Salt and pepper

½ cup ketchup

**UTENSILS NEEDED:**
Large bowl, sauté pan, loaf pan (about 5 ½" x 10 ½"), wooden spoon

1. Preheat oven to 375°F.

2. In a sauté pan, cook the onions, garlic, and carrots in oil until tender. Season with salt and pepper. Place in a large bowl to cool.

3. Add the rest of the ingredients when onions are cool, except the ketchup. Add salt and pepper. Mix well.

4. At this stage I sauté a ½ inch patty to check for seasoning before I cook the actual loaf. I cook it because, really, who wants to taste raw meat?

5. Once seasoned to your liking, place into a loaf pan. Top with ketchup and place into the oven.

6. Cook for approximately 25–30 minutes. Loaf will be firm to the touch. Stick a knife into the middle – if the knife comes out hot, the loaf is cooked through. The ketchup should be nice and caramelized.

7. Allow to rest for 5 minutes. Slice and serve.

You can use ground beef instead of turkey – just allow 10 more minutes to cook, as ground beef has more fat.

Put part of the meatloaf mixture into muffin cups and cook until done (less time than a whole loaf). These are great to freeze and send along in a lunchbox!

# Best Mashed Potatoes Ever

**GRAINS** **VEGGIES** **DAIRY** **EXTRAS**

---

*Prep Time: 20 minutes*    *Cook Time: 25 minutes*    *Yield: 6-8 servings*

---

6–8 Yukon Gold potatoes (about 4 pounds), peeled

1 stick very cold salted butter, cut into ½" cubes

Salt

½ - ¾ cup milk or heavy cream (Don't use skim milk – for the very best flavor, use real cream.)

**UTENSILS NEEDED:**
3-quart saucepan, rubber spatula, stand mixer or hand beater with whisk attachment, small saucepan

1. Dice the peeled potatoes into approximately 1-inch pieces. Make sure all the dices are a uniform size for even cooking.

2. Place the potatoes into the saucepan, cover with cold water (by two inches), and season with salt.

3. Bring to a boil over high heat. Once full boil is reached, reduce heat to a medium simmer. Cook until tender, about 15–20 minutes.

4. While the potatoes are cooking, heat the milk or heavy cream in a small saucepan just until it reaches a boil, then immediately take off the heat.

5. Drain potatoes and place in a bowl to mix with a whisk. If you have a stand mixer, use with the whisk attachment; if not, use a hand beater with a whisk attachment.

6. Turn the mixer on slow to medium speed, breaking down the potatoes. Scrape down the bowl as you go. Slowly add cubes of cold butter (this is called emulsifying – the cold butter is incorporated and blended into the hot potatoes). When all the butter is added, turn off the mixer and scrape down again.

7. Turn back on to slow speed, and add enough of the heated milk to reach the consistency your family likes.

8. Taste and adjust seasonings. Re-mix if you add seasoning. Serve.

## A WORD ON POTATOES:

Taste the water – it should have flavor. Seasoned water will flavor the potatoes in their raw state . This works better than adding salt to cooked potatoes, which won't absorb seasoning as effectively.

Use Yukon Gold potatoes; they have less starch and a creamier consistency.

When cooking potatoes, drain and mix immediately after they are done cooking. When potatoes sit in still water, they'll absorb the water. If you let the potatoes sit for too long after draining, they will become very gluteny and starchy, not fluffy.

Potatoes are one of those foods requiring immediacy. For very smooth potatoes, put the thoroughly mixed and emulsified potatoes through a food mill. Any remaining lumps will be gone. You can also add roasted garlic and fresh herbs when whisking the potatoes.

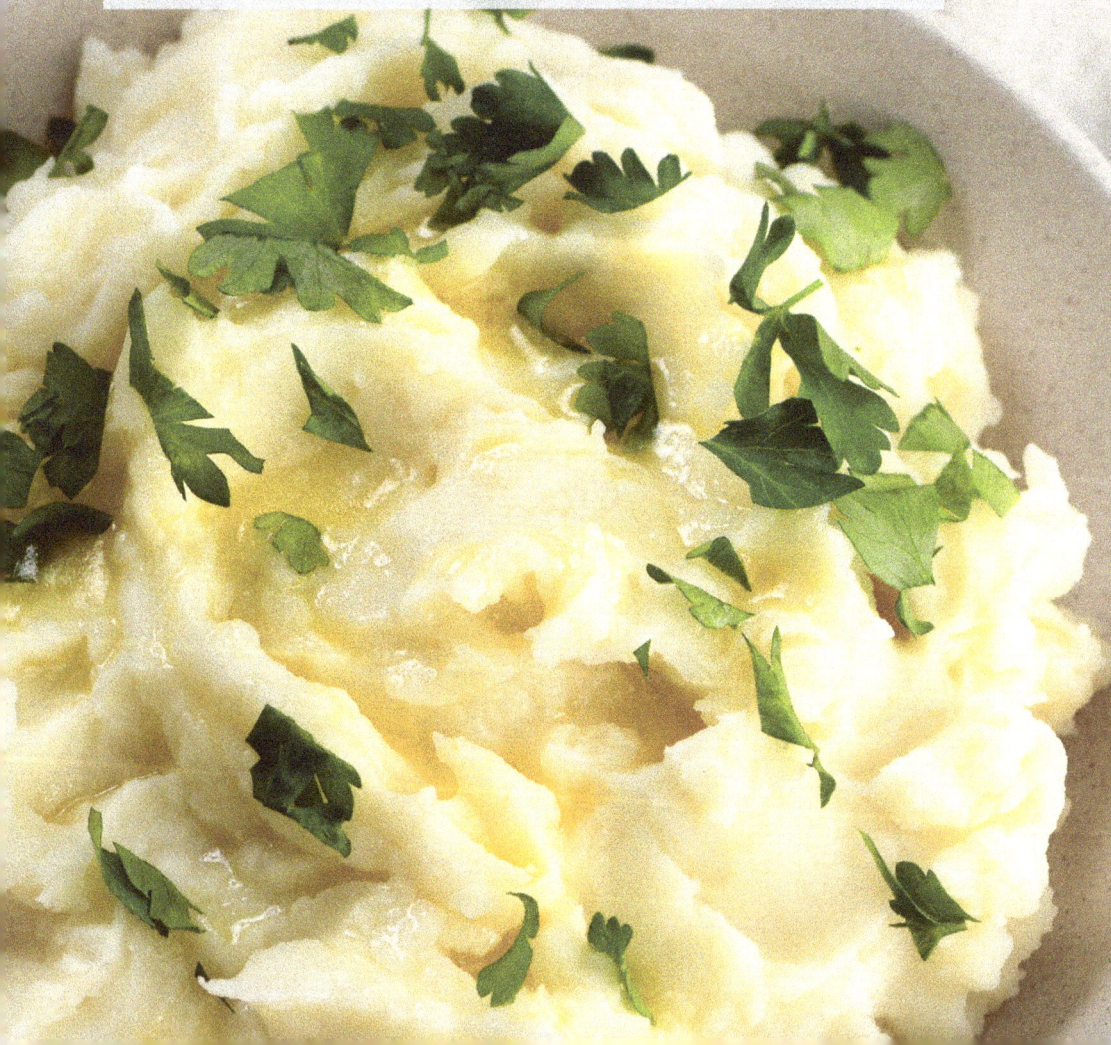

# Desserts & Treats

Save these lovely desserts for weekends or special occasions. Try to encourage fresh fruit for dessert. A small amount of fresh cream over some ripe peaches and blueberries is a wonderful treat! My grandmother was Danish, and they ate stinky cheese for dessert!

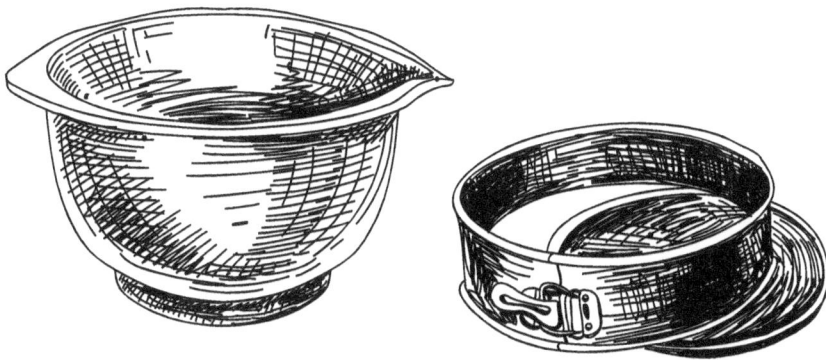

**FRUITS** **DAIRY** **PROTEIN** **EXTRAS**

# Lemon Curd ⟨WITH⟩ Blueberries

*Prep Time: 10 minutes*    *Cook Time: 15 minutes*    *Yield: 6-8 servings*

½ cup sugar

2 eggs

½ cup heavy cream

½ cup lemon juice

1 pint blueberries, fresh or frozen

2 Tablespoons cold butter

**UTENSILS NEEDED:**
Whisk, stainless steel pot

1. Place all ingredients except blueberries and cold butter into the saucepan.

2. Put on medium-high heat and whisk until thick (about 10 minutes). The mixture should coat the back of a spoon.

3. Remove from heat and whisk in the butter.

4. Chill lemon curd for at least an hour before serving.

5. Serve with blueberries (or just eat it straight out of the bowl, which is what I do sometimes when no one is looking).

You can make mini tarts by simply spooning some lemon curd into premade pie shells and adding a spoonful of blueberries (or raspberries, cherries, sliced strawberries – or a berry mix).

Follow with a dollop of fresh whipped cream, or just add a squirt from one of those aerosol cans – I'm very popular with my kids when I have one of those on hand, because they each usually get some straight from the can as well.

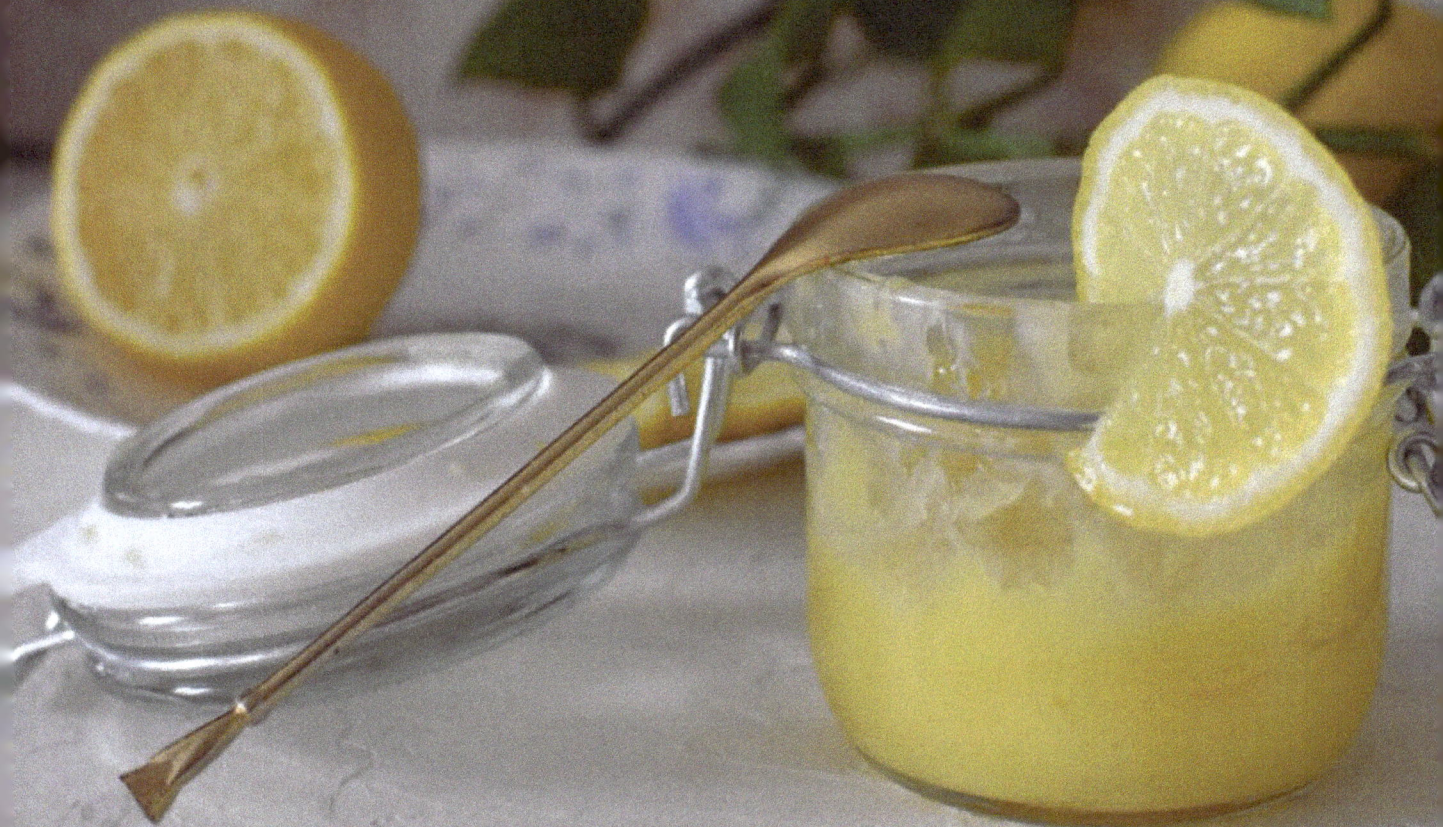

# Grilled Fruits

*Prep Time: 10 minutes*    *Cook Time: 15 minutes*    *Yield: 6-8 servings*

2 peaches, pitted and cut into eighths

1 fresh pineapple, sliced ½" thick

Fresh cherries

2 Fuji apples (seeded and cored), cut into eighths

2 Bosc pears (seeded and cored), cut into eighths

1 teaspoon vanilla extract

2 Tablespoons olive oil

Pinch of sea salt

Fresh ground pepper (maybe only for the big kids)

**UTENSILS NEEDED:**
Grill brush, tongs, sheet tray, cloth to oil grill, large bowl, grill basket

1. Pre-heat your grill. Great if you've prepared dinner on it already – just clean it off so your fruit doesn't taste like chicken!

2. Place all fruit in a large bowl. Add oil, vanilla, and season with pinch of salt. Toss to coat all fruit.

3. Wipe grill with oiled cloth. Place fruits on the grill or in a grill basket for smaller fruit. Rotate after a minute or so to make grill marks.

4. Turn over after 4 minutes and cook on the opposite side. You want them to be a bit al dente (firm) or else they will turn to mush on the grill.

5. Use tongs to remove from grill and place on a sheet tray. Mix together (if fruits are too large, cut down to bite-sized pieces). Arrange on a plate and enjoy.

Alternatively, you can roast the fruits on a tray in the oven at 400°F for approximately 15–20 minutes.

# Flourless Chocolate Cake
## ⟨WITH⟩ Fresh Raspberries

*Prep Time: 20 min.   Cook Time: 20-25 min.   Yield: 10-12 servings (20 cupcakes)*

12 ounces bittersweet chocolate

12 ounces salted butter

1 ½ cup organic granulated sugar

12 egg yolks

10 egg whites

Cupcake liners

Cooking spray

**UTENSILS NEEDED:**
Stand mixer with bowl and whip attachment (or handheld mixer), saucepan with small bowl (double boiler), rubber spatula, cupcake tins or ½ sheet tray/cookie sheet

1. Preheat oven to 375°F.

2. Start by melting the chocolate, butter, and sugar in a double boiler. (If you don't have one, just use a saucepan filled halfway with water with a small bowl on top. Bring to a boil, then reduce to medium heat.) When melted, remove from heat and let cool.

3. In a stand mixer fitted with wire whip (or with hand mixer), whip egg yolks until they are big and fluffy (about 10 min). Pour into a large bowl and set aside.

4. Thoroughly wash and dry mixer bowl. Add egg whites and whip to their fullest (white fluffy clouds), approximately 5 minutes. Add egg whites to egg yolks using rubber spatula. Be gentle – try not to break down the fluffiness.

5. Add cooled chocolate and sugar mixture. Fold together gently to blend all ingredients. Spray pans with cooking spray or use cupcake liners. Pour into cupcake tins and fill ¾ way or pour onto greased ½ sheet tray.

6. Bake approximately 12–15 minutes at 375°F. Will be moist in the middle. Serve warm with fresh raspberries.

You can use semisweet chocolate – just use 1 cup of sugar. Substitute other favorite fruits. Whip some fresh cream with a hint of vanilla. Sprinkle a little powdered sugar on top.

# Vando's Oatmeal Raisin Cookies

GRAINS | FRUITS | DAIRY | EXTRAS

*Prep Time: 15 minutes    Cook Time: 20-30 minutes    Yield: 2 dozen 2 ounce cookies*

---

2 ¼ cups oats (either quick cooking or Irish, although 100% whole grain quick oats will work best)

½ pound cold butter, cubed (2 sticks)

¾ cup sugar

¾ cup brown sugar

1 teaspoon vanilla

2 eggs

1 ¼ cup organic all-purpose flour (try a 50/50 mixture of whole wheat and white)

1 teaspoon baking soda

1 ½ cups raisins

**UTENSILS NEEDED:**
Cookie sheets, stand mixer with bowl and paddle (or handheld mixer), rubber spatula

1. Preheat oven to 350°F.

2. Use mixer to cream together butter, sugars, and vanilla with paddle attachment on medium speed.

3. When blended, add the eggs; continue to mix on medium until eggs are blended in.

4. Slowly add the flour, baking soda, and oats.

5. Scrape down the bowl with a rubber spatula. Add the raisins and blend carefully on low to incorporate.

6. You can refrigerate the dough at this point until it's cold. Cold dough forms better cookies.

7. Place 2-ounce scoops of the dough on the cookie sheet, spacing the cookies out by one inch.

8. Bake for about 12–15 minutes.

9. Remove from oven and allow to cool.

10. Serve on a nice plate – if they actually last long enough to plate them.

I usually measure my dry ingredients onto waxed paper, then make a cone out of the wax paper and, with the mixer on low, sort of slide the dry ingredients into the batter.

# Peach–Cherry Cobbler

*Prep Time: 10 minutes* | *Cook Time: 20 minutes* | *Yield: 10-12 servings*

4 cups of fresh sliced peaches or 32 ounces frozen sliced peaches

2 cups fresh pitted cherries or 16 ounces frozen cherries

¼ cup melted butter

1 teaspoon vanilla

¼ cup organic brown sugar

½ cup all-purpose flour

16 ounces canned large biscuits

**UTENSILS NEEDED:**
Casserole dish (8" x 8"), bowl

1. Preheat oven to 400°F. Place fruit in a bowl and add the flour, butter, vanilla, and sugar, and toss until coated.

2. Place in a buttered or greased casserole dish and top with canned biscuits, making sure the biscuits are evenly spaced. Sprinkle a little brown sugar on top.

3. Bake at 400°F for 15 minutes or until biscuits are nicely golden brown.

4. Serve with vanilla ice cream or whipped cream.

**Try different fruit mixtures: apple and cherry, peach and blueberry, peach and mango or pear.**

GRAINS  FRUITS  EXTRAS

# Banana Bread

*Prep Time: 15 minutes*    *Cook Time: 60 minutes*    *Yield: 10-12 servings*

1 ¼ stick butter

½ cup brown sugar

½ cup granulated organic sugar

1 teaspoon vanilla

3 very ripe bananas, mashed

1 teaspoon ground cinnamon

¼ teaspoon salt

2 eggs

2 cups 50/50 organic flour (half wheat, half white)

1 teaspoon baking soda

1 teaspoon baking powder

¼ cup sour cream

Butter for greasing the pan

**UTENSILS NEEDED:**
Stand mixer with paddle (or mixing bowl and beaters), 5 ½" x 10 ½" loaf pan, rubber spatula

1. Preheat oven to 350°F. Grease and sugar loaf pan.

2. In the bowl of the stand mixer, cream together the butter, sugars, and vanilla. Scrape down the bowl.

3. Add the bananas, cinnamon, salt, and eggs. Continue mixing for 1 minute.

4. Add the flour, baking soda, and baking powder, and mix at low speed for 2 minutes.

5. Add sour cream and scrape down the bowl. Mix until blended.

6. Pour into the prepared loaf pan. Sprinkle a little sugar on top to ensure a crispy outside and moist inside.

7. Bake for 60 minutes, rotating after 30 minutes. A toothpick inserted into the center should come out clean.

8. Remove from the oven and let cool for 15 minutes before serving.

You can freeze bananas when they get too ripe and use them for this recipe, but make sure you thaw them first and do not use any of the water that comes out – just the banana pulp itself.

Try adding ½ cup toasted chopped walnuts or any other favorite nut, dried fruits, or sliced maraschino cherries.

# Activities

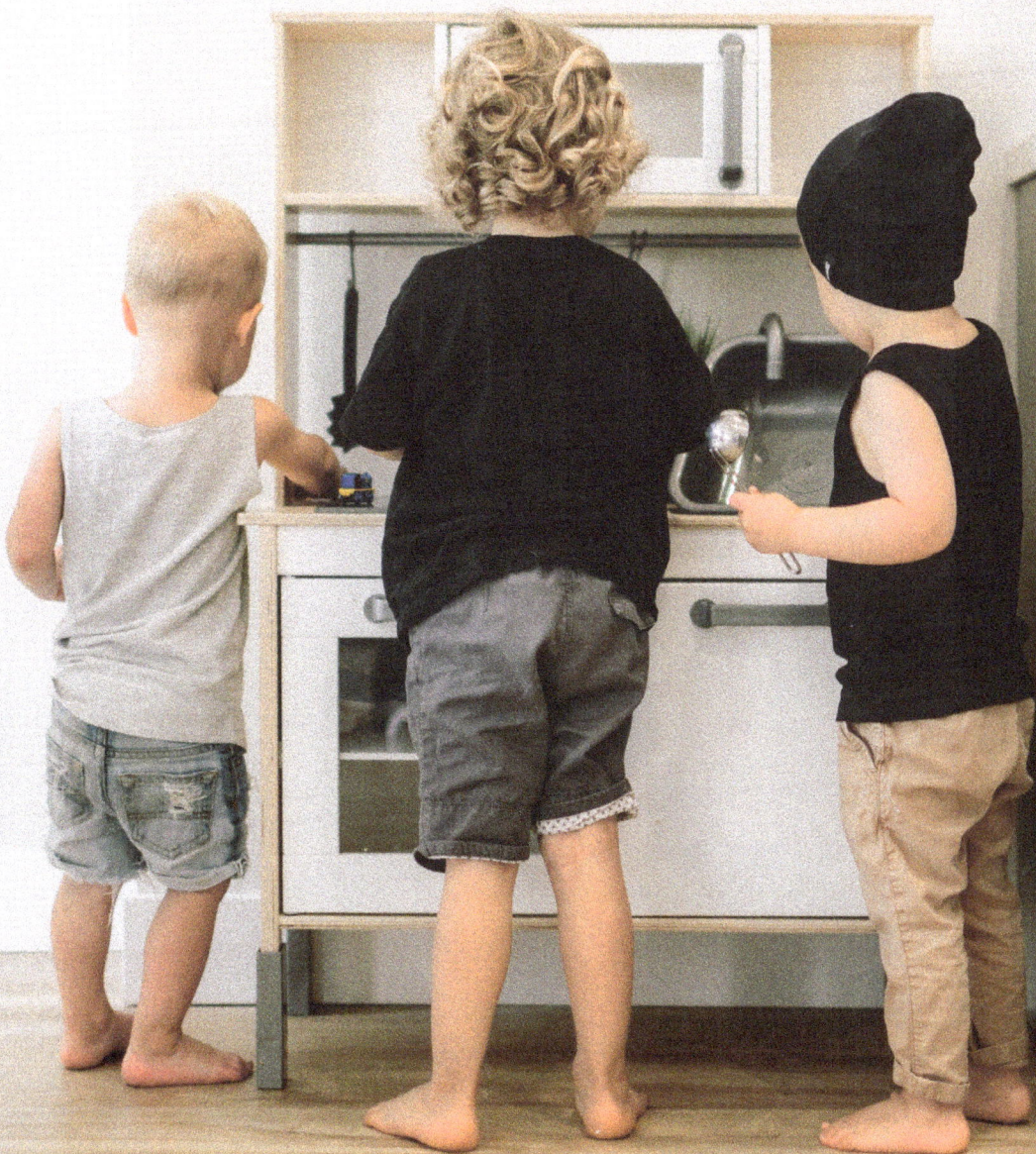

# Old School P.E.

It's time to get moving! All the nutrition training in the world won't stick unless your kids are active. When we get moving, we feel better and crave less.

Coach Brookins served as the awesome P.E. coach at our local elementary school. He has been encouraging kids to stay active for many years, and when asked to contribute ways to keep our kids moving, he jumped on board! His Old School P.E. activities are designed to get your kids (and you!) moving while having fun.

## Coach Brookins' Philosophy on Exercise

- Breathe.

- Keep it simple. Make it as fun as possible. Make it a part of your life.

- Give yourself short breaks from exercise. This will help you avoid burning out and give your body time to re-energize, recuperate, and revitalize.

- Include loved ones in exercise plans.

- Plan on it being a bit of work, but know that it will definitely have a big payoff – mind, body, and soul.

- Set realistic short-term goals, then revisit and reset those goals on a regular basis, such as 2-4 week intervals.

- Count active playtime as exercise. Adults should not be afraid to relax and act like a crazy chicken sometimes too!

- Plan family outings to the park or to watch sporting events – learning about and watching different sports can be a motivator for your own exercise and activity levels.

- Never make exercise painful. Discomfort is an indication that you should slow it down a bit or take a rest.

- NEVER use activity as a punishment!

- Put a spin on the above and make activity/exercise a reward for doing chores, good school reports, eating well, etc. "You've done a great job today! We can go for a bike ride after dinner."

- Do not stereotype yourself or anyone else as an "athlete," "naturally fit," or anything of that sort. Everyone's body craves activity and exercise, and with a bit of patience (and putting your ego on standby for a while) EVERYONE is capable of being good at exercise!

- Do some COMMERCIAL-CIZE! Train your kids to move while they watch TV. Get up and move during the commercials. Walk up and down the stairs, or do some of the great exercises in here – just get moving. (Added benefit: they won't see 100 sugary cereal commercials.)

- Be a good role model!

# Walkin' the Dog
## *(straddle hand walks)*

1. Stand with your feet apart – wider than your shoulders, knees slightly bent, hands on hips.

2. Bend over at your waist, placing both hands flat on the floor slightly in front of your feet.

3. Leaving your feet in place (try to keep your heels down), walk your hands forward on the floor for six (6) steps.

4. Pause for four (4) counts then walk your hands backward six (6) steps.

5. Raise upright and put your hands on your hips, making sure that you maintain a straight posture.

6. Pause for four (4) counts.

## Repeat for 5–10 repetitions.

Stop immediately if it's painful. Stretches should always be comfortable.

**Age Group:**
4+

**How Long It Takes:**
5–10 minutes

**How Many People:**
1+

**Equipment Needed:**
None

**Space Needed:**
4' x 4' floor space

# Sofa Dips
## *(or chair dips)*

1. Stand in front of a sofa.

2. Squat down in front of the sofa, facing away from it.

3. Place the palms of your hands on the edge of the sofa with your fingers hanging off (make sure it won't move if you push on it!).

4. With arms slightly bent, walk both feet out in front of you until your legs are straight. Your weight will be resting on your hands and your heels.

5. Slowly lower yourself down by bending your elbows. Try to lower yourself more each time.

## Do 6 repetitions, then rest and repeat.

**Excellent to do while watching TV!**

**Age Group:**
8+

**How Long It Takes:**
5–10 minutes

**How Many People:**
1+

**Equipment Needed:**
Sofa or 2 chairs (that won't move)

**Space Needed:**
6 feet in front of sofa

# Couch Press

## *(sofa push-ups)*

1. Kneel down, facing the sofa. Put your hands on the edge of the seat, about shoulder width apart.

2. Raise your knees and walk your feet back away from the sofa. Try to get your body, legs, and head in a straight line. Support your weight on your toes and with your arms.

3. Keeping your back straight, lower and raise your body by bending your elbows.

## Repeat up to 12 times. Do 3 or 4 sets.

A challenging variation to this activity is to put your toes on the sofa and your hands on the floor, keeping your back straight. Try not to fall on your nose!

**Age Group:**
8+

**How Long It Takes:**
5–10 minutes

**How Many People:**
1+

**Equipment Needed:**
1 sofa (that won't move)

**Space Needed:**
6 feet in front of sofa

# Crab Dips
*(reverse push-ups)*

1. Sit on the floor.

2. Place your hands on the floor on each side of your body, fingers pointing towards your feet.

3. Bend your knees and keep your feet flat on the floor.

4. Keep your shoulders in line with your hands and your feet in line with your knees as much as possible.

5. Raise your midsection off the floor.

6. Slowly bend your elbows and lower your upper body down towards the floor 2–4 inches.

7. Slowly push your body up again until your arms are extended straight.

8. Repeat until fatigued.

**Do 2–4 sets. Use your stomach muscles to hold your midsection off the floor.**

**Age Group:**
4+

**How Long It Takes:**
2–5 minutes

**How Many People:**
1+

**Equipment Needed:**
None

**Space Needed:**
4' x 4'

# Chop Sticks
*(leg raises)*

1. Lie down on your back.

2. Place your hands beside your bottom to support your back, if needed. Once you get really strong, you can put them out to the side or above your head.

3. With legs straight and stomach muscles tight, raise both feet 12–18 inches off the floor. Gently tap your heels together, pretending that you are grabbing something with chopsticks!

4. Slowly lower both feet back to the floor (try moving your feet 1 inch per second, counting aloud).

## Repeat 6–12 times.

5. Next: Turn over on one side. Your body can be slightly bent at the hips. Put your lower arm straight under your head or support your head with your hand. Place your top hand in front of you to prevent your body from rolling forward.

6. With legs straight and stomach muscles tight, lift your top leg 12–18 inches off the floor.

7. Slowly lower your leg, pacing as described above.

## Repeat the exercise 6–12 times, then repeat on the other side.

**Age Group:**
3+

**How Long It Takes:**
5–10 minutes

**How Many People:**
1+

**Equipment Needed:**
None

**Space Needed:**
Open floor space

# Helicopter
## *(march & trunk twist)*

1. March in place by lifting your knees high (90° or until the top part of your leg is flat), letting your foot hang down. Do this 20 times while you swing your arms back and forth. Get your march on!

2. Stop – extend your arms to the sides and bend slightly at the knees.

3. SLOWLY twist your trunk at the waist, trying to turn your shoulders to the right side. Return to front and repeat to the left side.

4. Do 10 trunk twists in total.

**Repeat from the very beginning 3–6 times. Concentrate on breathing in and out.**

**Age Group:**
3+

**How Long It Takes:**
5–10 minutes

**How Many People:**
1+

**Equipment Needed:**
None

**Space Needed:**
4' x 4'

# Hi-Yah!

## *(squat kicks)*

**LOWER BODY STRENGTH & COORDINATION**

1. Stand upright with your feet shoulder width apart and arms extended to the side.

2. Slowly squat down, lowering your bottom towards the floor. Try to keep your knees over your feet.

3. Stand up and kick your right foot forward, then your left foot forward. (Keep in mind you aren't moving anywhere, just standing in place and kicking.)

## Repeat 8–12 times.

Don't kick too hard, or you'll pop out a knee!

**Age Group:**
4+

**How Long It Takes:**
5–10 minutes

**How Many People:**
1+

**Equipment Needed:**
None

**Space Needed:**
Open floor space

# Chicken Wings

## *(arm stretch & arm circles)*

1. Stand with your legs shoulder width apart, arms out to the side. Point your right elbow towards the sky, with your right hand touching between your shoulder blades.

2. Bring your left hand over your head, and gently pull your right elbow backwards. You should feel a comfortable stretch in the back of your arm.

3. Repeat with other arm.

4. Straighten both arms out to the side.

5. Make big circles forward. Try to do 15 circles.

6. Make big circles backwards. Try to do 15, and work your way up when you can.

## Repeat from the stretches 3 times.

**Age Group:**
4+

**How Long It Takes:**
5–10 minutes

**How Many People:**
1+

**Equipment Needed:**
None

**Space Needed:**
Open floor space

# Dictionary Press

1. Lie on your back. Hold a dictionary with both hands above your chest.

2. Use your hands to press it upwards, extending your arms straight, and then back down to your chest, 8–16 times.

3. Rest briefly. Open the dictionary to a random page and read the definition of three words.

## Perform 2 more sets, resting briefly in between.

**Age Group:**
6+

**How Long It Takes:**
5–10 minutes

**How Many People:**
1+

**Equipment Needed:**
Dictionary

**Space Needed:**
Open floor space

# Sit-'n-Catch

If a softball is not available, tie a piece of fabric (shirt, towel, etc.) into a couple of knots.

1. Kid #1 sits on the floor in a sit-up position with knees bent.

2. Kid #2 stands a few feet away, facing Kid #1.

3. Kid #2 tosses the ball/fabric to Kid #1 just above head level.

4. Kid #1 catches the ball and slowly rolls down to the ground – while holding the ball above their head – and touches the ball to the floor.

5. Kid #1 slowly sits back up with the ball still above their head and tosses the ball back to Kid #2.

## Repeat 6-12 times.

6. Kid #1 and #2 switch places and continue the exercise. The exercise is done when both partners have completed 2–4 sets of this activity.

**Age Group:**
6+

**How Long It Takes:**
5–10 minutes

**How Many People:**
2

**Equipment Needed:**
Ball or a tied up ball of fabric

**Space Needed:**
4' x 8'

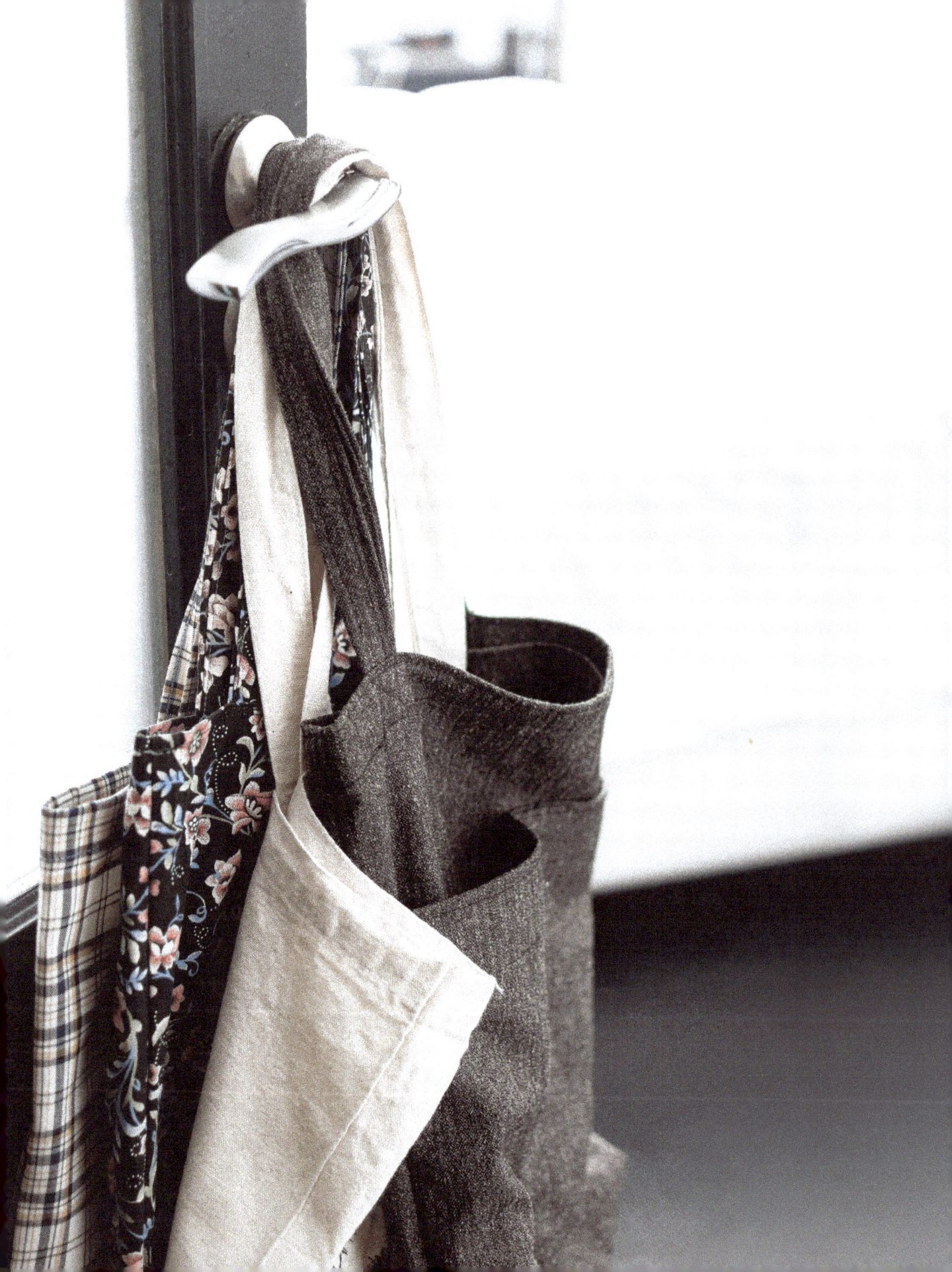

# Pantry Parade
## *(lunges)*

1. Clear floor space and choose items to put in a bag that can be comfortably carried in one hand.

2. Grip the bag in one hand. Stand with your feet together, facing the clear floor space.

3. Take a giant step forward with your left foot and touch your right knee to the floor, pausing for 2–4 seconds while maintaining balance. (Try to keep your front knee over your foot.)

4. Leaving the left foot in place, rise up and step forward with the right foot, bringing it alongside the left foot.

5. Repeat with right foot first.

6. Continue alternating right and left steps, while maintaining a comfortable grip on the bag, for 6 steps.

## Repeat the activity 2–6 times.

Having to maintain balance while holding the bag forces you to also work your body's core muscles. Alternate the side on which you hold the weighted bag.

This exercise may also be done without carrying any weights.

**Age Group:**
6+

**How Long It Takes:**
5–10 minutes

**How Many People:**
1+

**Equipment Needed:**
Grocery bag, weighted items (cans, toys, packaged foods, dumbbells)

**Space Needed:**
Hallway or 8–10 feet of unobstructed floor space

**STRENGTH, BALANCE, & COOPERATION**

# Statue Pose Duel

1. Kid #1 does a statue pose. Anything is great – try to make it a bit difficult to balance. Hold the pose for a 10 count.

2. If Kid #1 is successful, then Kid #2 must also hold the identical pose for 10 seconds.

3. Each participant takes turns challenging each other to a pose.

## In order to score a point, you must successfully complete your pose and your opponent must be unsuccessful in completing your pose.

**Age Group:**
4+

**How Long It Takes:**
10–20 minutes (try them during the commercials if you are watching TV!)

**How Many People:**
2

**Equipment Needed:**
None

**Space Needed:**
Open floor space

# Dice-ercize

1. Write down a list of exercises on a piece of paper. Choose an order among the participants (such as youngest to oldest or clockwise around a circle).

2. Participant #1 chooses an exercise.

3. Participant # 1 then rolls the dice and adds them up. All participants perform the rolled number of the chosen exercise.

4. Participant #2 repeats steps 2 and 3, and so on.

## Add, subtract, or multiply the dice.

If all else doesn't work out, this may increase math skills!

**Age Group:**
6+

**How Long It Takes:**
10–20+ minutes

**How Many People:**
2+

**Equipment Needed:**
Paper, pair of dice

**Space Needed:**
Open space

# Coin Toss Fitness

1. On one piece of paper, draw a large grid with 6 boxes. Allow each participant to choose at least one activity/ exercise to write in each box.

2. On the other piece of paper, draw another large grid with 6 boxes and number the boxes by twos (2–12).

3. Choose an order among participants.

4. The first participant tosses one coin on the exercise paper and the other coin on the numbered paper.

5. All of the remaining participants must perform the exercises, with the repetition selected by the coin toss (such as 6 helicopters).

6. The next participant tosses the coins, and the game continues.

**Age Group:**
5+

**How Long It Takes:**
10–20+ minutes

**How Many People:**
2+

**Equipment Needed:**
2 pieces of paper, pen or pencil, 2 coins

**Space Needed:**
Open floor space

# Drama-cize

We asked Amy Handler, who taught creative movement and drama at our local elementary school, to put together some great activities that involve a little more drama. These "Drama-cizes" are her specialty! A little bit different than the physical exercises in the previous section, these activities will spark imagination and get your kids moving in new and different ways.

We asked Ms. Handler to tailor some so that they can be performed while in front of the TV (they might as well be using their brain!) and some to be done while riding in the car. In an emergency, you can use any of these – anywhere. They just might lead to some of your most hilarious family memories!

## Did you know your imagination is a muscle?

Kids learn better when they are having fun and being active, and pretending is how children learn about the world around them. Some deal, huh? Kids get to pretend, be silly, use their imaginations, all while becoming better adjusted to their world, enhancing self-esteem, building communication and problem solving skills, and getting exercise – without even knowing it. All they think they are doing is having fun and getting some sillies out.

So why not use creative play to turn everyday activities into superfun adventures? Who knew there was more than one way to set the table, or that a long car trip can become much more than the quintessential "Are we there yet?"

Looking for a new way to remove your potatoes from the couch? We've provided many silly ideas to help them rev up their imaginations. They'll be having so much fun, they'll forget what program they're missing. Or, if they have to watch, we've provided some great ways to make it a bit more creative and active.

# Meal Movies

Are your kids starving before their dinner is ready? Are they asking to eat hot fudge sundaes for dinner? Have they eaten you out of house and home, and they're still hungry? Let your kids create their own personal, internal movies of their greatest eating conquest.

1.  Have your "starving" child close their eyes and imagine their favorite thing to eat, their most unhealthy craving, or what they ate for dinner that they want more of. They need to really concentrate with all of their senses.

2.  How does the food look? Have them imagine every detail of the food, down to how many chocolate chips are in their muffin or how many slices of lettuce on their sandwich.

3.  How does the food smell? Make sure they can imagine its aroma before they bite into it.

4.  What does the food taste like? How does it make their body move when it tastes good?

5.  What about the feel? How does it feel against their lips and tongue? How easy is it to swallow and chew? Do they feel it against their teeth as it crunches?

6.  How does it sound? Can they hear it crunch or squish? What noises do their mouths make as they chew?

Once they have played this movie in their head, they can act it out for you. Have them really focus on it. Try not to laugh or think of anything else.

If time is still draggin', have them create a second "movie" of something they don't like eating. They can even challenge each other to a rousing game of charades – what are they eating?

**Age Group:**
4+

**How Long It Takes:**
10 minutes

**How Many People:**
1+

**Equipment Needed:**
Only a great imagination

**Space Needed:**
Just as much space as your child/children take up

# Mealmaking Mirror

Want to involve your kids in the cooking but you're too afraid of their knife-throwing abilities? Or do you just not have enough time to get them too involved? Try teaching your child our patented cooking techniques.

1.  Have your child closely observe what you are doing – from the way you hold your knife, to which way you squint when you hold up your measuring cup for accuracy, to how you wipe your hands on your apron.

2.  Now it's their job to copy every detail of what you are doing – they must only pretend to see, feel, and touch all the food and tools. They are your cooking mirror, and should be doing everything you are.

3.  At the end of the process they will have a beautiful, healthy, home-cooked "meal" that tastes as great as yours.

Don't forget to have them look for every single movement detail. Make sure they really observe you, rather than just anticipating what you will do.

You could play this once you are at the table too – switching leaders and pretending to eat like them, but this time they can use real food instead of just their imagination.

**Age Group:**
4+

**How Long It Takes:**
Time to cook a meal, or as long as their attentions will span

**How Many People:**
1+

**Equipment Needed:**
Only whatever you're doing in the kitchen. Your kids need nothing – that's the point!

**Space Needed:**
Enough room in your kitchen to not get jostled by their movements

# Dramatic Recipe Readings

Instead of springing for one of those cookbook holders or running back and forth to your recipe, employ your child to help you read it.

1. Challenge your kid to read the recipe instructions so you can hear them very clearly.

2. Once they can do that with confidence, add some drama. Ask them to read it in all sorts of different ways – as loud as they can, as quiet as they can, like a famous movie star, as if they are scared to give you the information, as if it's a burning secret, with a French accent, the list can go on and on...

You can carry this one out by letting them help serve the meal, taking on one of these new identities/qualities.

If their reading capabilities aren't quite there, then feed them some lines.

**Age Group:**
7+ (or whenever your child becomes a fluent reader)

**How Long It Takes:**
As long as it takes to cook your meal

**How Many People:**
1+

**Equipment Needed:**
A loud voice and a recipe

**Space Needed:**
Just as much space as your kids take up

# How Many Robots Does It Take to Set the Table?

Make setting the family meal table fun and active by taking on different roles as you do it. You can be robots, bandits, rock stars, pirates, or chickens as you put all the plates and cups into their proper places.

1. Choose your character. Think about how your character would move – how do they hold their bodies differently than you do? How would they talk? Can you change your voice to talk more like your character?

2. After you change your voice, think about what they would say – do robots even know what a plate is? "Processing foreign object to be placed on eating surface." Do rock stars really know the proper place to put the knives and forks? "My road manager usually does this for me. I'll just put them here underneath the plate." Can chickens even reach the table? "Bok!"

3. Put your character into action and get to work actually setting the table.

If you can't agree what everyone should be, everyone can choose a different kind of character. You can see how these types interact while they are working. Maybe the rock star hires the robot to be their new personal assistant, or maybe the chicken pecks holes in the robot to cause it to short circuit.

**Age Group:**
4+

**How Long It Takes:**
10 minutes

**How Many People:**
1+

**Equipment Needed:**
A table and its settings – might want to save the good china for another night

**Space Needed:**
A kitchen/dining room

# Race Through Your Dinner
## *(This has nothing to do with eating in a hurry)*

Work off your dinner and make room for dessert as you relay race with your family through different foods.

1. Think about the foods you are eating. What would it feel like to move through an entire room full of them? Really pretend that you are racing through jello, mashed potatoes, salad dressing, hot coffee, cold water, or even a school of salmon.

2. Choose your first food to race through.

3. On your mark, get set, GO!

4. Pick a new food and repeat.

It's really important to remember this isn't an actual get-there-first kind of race. It's not about how fast you move but how well you adapt your movements. Make others see you would actually slosh through mashed potatoes!

It will help if you remember to use your whole body to really feel these foods all around you. How does that change how fast or slow you move? How do you hold your body?

Try keeping these movements going while eating dinner – move like you are moving through the food you are eating while you eat it.

**Age Group:**
4+

**How Long It Takes:**
20 minutes

**How Many People:**
2+

**Equipment Needed:**
None

**Space Needed:**
Open space

# Kitchen Props

Did you know that a frying pan makes a great magnifying glass? Or that an egg beater is the exact same shape as a microphone? Ever use a loaf of French bread as a sword? Use your imagination to give everyday kitchen objects other silly uses.

1. Choose your first item from what you see in the kitchen. Make sure it's not dirty, dangerous, or in use.

2. Pass it back and forth between yourselves, coming up with different unconventional uses for it.

3. Make sure you show what it is with dialogue. "I can't quite get this motorboat going" (eggbeater), instead of just saying, "It's a boat motor."

4. See how many different silly uses you can come up with for each object.

5. Pick a new item and repeat.

If you can't think of ideas, run through a list of categories in your head that it might be – an animal, clothing, food...

If you have lots of people, you can work in teams, going one team at a time.

**Age Group:**
7+

**How Long It Takes:**
10 minutes

**How Many People:**
2+

**Equipment Needed:**
Random kitchen items

**Space Needed:**
Open space

# TV Dance Party

Afraid to leave your TV set during commercials because you don't want to miss one tiny second of your favorite show? Turn lemons into lemonade by turning those boring commercials into the greatest dance party ever!

1. Whenever it seems like your show is about to stop for a commercial, stand up and get ready to move and groove.

2. Start dancing as wildly as you can all through the commercials.

3. Use your reflexes to stop and freeze immediately when they end.

4. Relax and enjoy your show until the next ad break.

5. Move as big and as crazily as you can, but don't forget to be looking out for the end of the commercial. You must freeze right away!

6. Take turns being the director, and call out what kind of dance party you will have during each break. Maybe the first one is a wiggle dance, the next one an on-the-floor dance, the next a dance-on-one-foot dance, etc.

**Age Group:**
3+

**How Long It Takes:**
About 5 minutes each break

**How Many People:**
1+

**Equipment Needed:**
A TV

**Space Needed:**
Open space

# Become Your Favorite TV Characters

Always wanted to be on TV, but you just can't seem to get out of your house and you don't have bus fare to Hollywood anyway? Try this activity and you'll be a star in your own living room.

1.  When your favorite show comes on, watch the opening credits where they introduce all the characters.

2.  Choose who you are going to be for the entire show.

3.  Every time your character comes on screen, copy their movements.

4.  Make sure you stay safe – you will have to be creative to figure out how you can pretend to do what a cartoon character does.

5.  If what they are doing is too tricky, you could try giving your character a signature move instead. Choose a movement that you think shows their personality. Every time they come on the screen, you must do this movement until they exit.

6.  OR, if they are on screen the whole time and you are getting tired, try doing their movement every time they talk instead.

**Age Group:**
5+

**How Long It Takes:**
As long as a TV show

**How Many People:**
1+

**Equipment Needed:**
A TV

**Space Needed:**
Open space

# Car Stories

Tired of hearing/saying, "Are we there yet?" Create stories together that are compelling enough to make them want to stay in the car forever.

1. Your story starts like so: "One day our family decided to take the car on a trip to the beach (or wherever it is you might be headed), when suddenly..."

2. The first player now has a chance to turn the story into something silly and fantastical. They must come up with something untrue that turns the trip into a wild adventure. "When suddenly their car lifted from the road and became a rocket on its way to Mars," or "When all the other cars on the road became wild dinosaurs that tried to eat them." They need only give one sentence.

3. The next player must continue with the given storyline and add to it, also only giving one sentence.

4. Continue in this manner until you get there, the story has a natural ending, or the group decides they want to start a new one.

Really listen to what the other players have contributed. If they say a pack of wild dogs were hitchhiking and demanded to get in your car, you must use that and take it further.

**Age Group:**
5+

**How Long It Takes:**
As long as it needs to, can go on forever

**How Many People:**
2+

**Equipment Needed:**
None

**Space Needed:**
The inside of a car

You might say, "And once they got in, they turned into wild monkeys," or "And we wouldn't let them in, but they scratched the door down." An example of not taking their story further might be: "And then I ate ice cream," or "And then we all landed on the moon."

Try not to think too much about what you think should happen before it's your turn – then you'll be thinking about your own idea instead of the story. If you aren't listening and use your idea anyway, the story might not make sense anymore.

If the stories get too long, rambling, or confusing, a parent can choose a time to say, "Find a way to end it in your next turn."

You could make your stories about what happens when you get to your destination or really anything you want, letting someone pick a new start each time.

For a bigger challenge, try the same thing but with each player only using one word at a time. It's much harder, but can get some even sillier results.

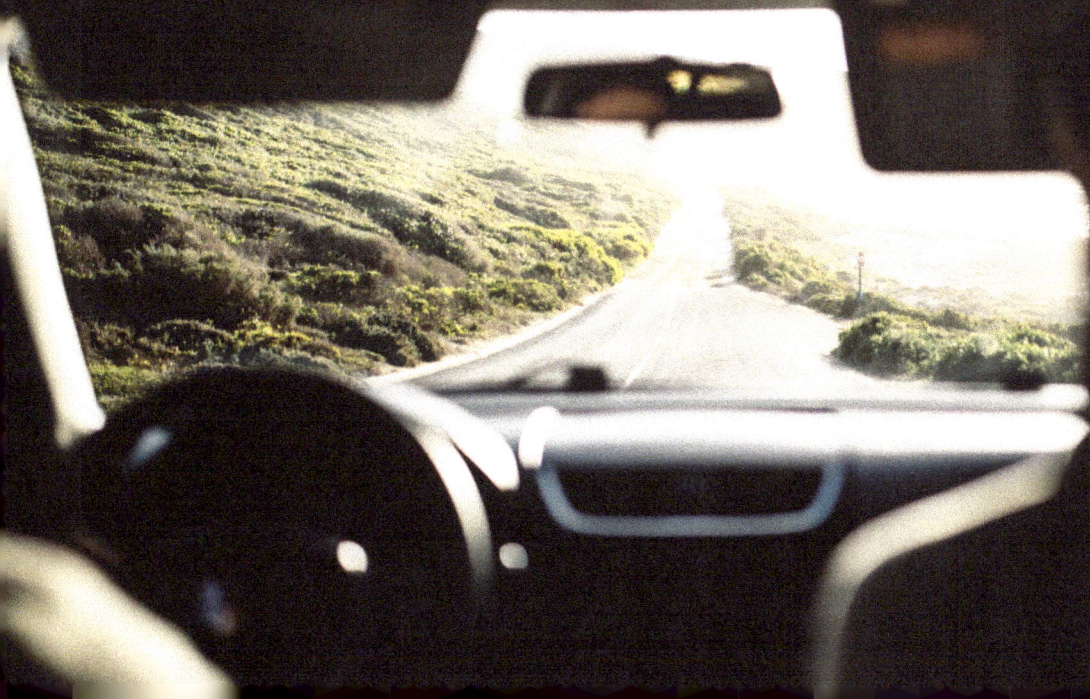

# Sit and Stand

Ever notice how many times people on TV change positions? Now you will, since you will be doing it with them.

1. When your show starts, watch every single character in the room. Watch for when one of them changes from sitting to standing or vice versa.

2. Every time they change positions, you change too.

3. If more than one character sits or stands in a row, you must change your position to a different way of sitting or standing.

4. Take a break during commercials and lay down. Or, if you aren't tired, do the same for the people on the commercials too.

5. There are about a billion ways to sit and stand. Don't get locked into just a few ways – really use your imagination to choose a new position each time.

6. You could also do this more like a mirror, where you choose one character to follow and sit and stand with them the whole time. But it's lots more fun to follow a bunch of people at once.

You can make it even more active and assign a different movement for sitting and standing (i.e., every time someone sits you jump, and every time someone stands you run in place).

**Age Group:**
5+

**How Long It Takes:**
As long as a TV show

**How Many People:**
1+

**Equipment Needed:**
A TV

**Space Needed:**
Open space

# When I Go To...

Use your imagination and memory on a long trip to help you flex your imagination and memory muscle.

1. The opening line is always: "When I go to (fill in the blank for wherever you are going), I am going to bring..."

2. The first player will name an item to bring. It can be something they actually brought on their trip or something completely silly and made up, which, of course, is the more fun option. "When I go to New York, I am going to bring a giant sack of 6-inch-long twigs."

3. The next player must repeat the opening line and then the first player's named item. Then they add their own item to the list. "When I go to New York, I am going to bring a giant sack of 6-inch-long twigs and a purple alien."

4. The following player must repeat everything said, plus their own item. "When I go to New York, I am going to bring a giant sack of 6-inch-long twigs, a purple alien, and my dog's water bowl."

Continue adding items to the list – see how long a list you can memorize.

You could make your answers have to fit into certain categories – things you would take to the beach, gross foods, favorite books, etc.

**Age Group:**
5+

**How Long It Takes:**
As long as it needs to, can go on forever

**How Many People:**
2+

**Equipment Needed:**
None

**Space Needed:**
The inside of a car

# Make Your Own Tongue Twisters

Tired of selling seashells by the seashore or woodchucks chucking wood? Now's your chance to remake the classics while giving your tongue and imagination a great workout.

1. Pick a letter that your group tongue twister is going to start with.

2. Have each player secretly pick a word that starts with that letter.

3. Go around the car one at a time and each say your word. Do this a few times, getting faster and faster until you can remember the words in order.

4. Take turns each saying the whole thing alone. Once you've really got it, say it as fast as you can three times in a row.

Try it in rounds, with each person starting theirs on the second word, third word, etc.

See how soft and loud you can say it. Try other variations too – fake crying, holding your tongue, plugging your nose, with an accent, etc.

**Age Group:**
6+

**How Long It Takes:**
As long as it needs to, can go on forever

**How Many People:**
2+

**Equipment Needed:**
None

**Space Needed:**
The inside of a car or anywhere

Getting
Everyone on
Board

# We All Need a Little Help!

Many families have help with their children at some point in their lives. No matter how much time we spend with our kids, they will come under the wing of other adults and educators at some point. Whether through a preschool, daycare, babysitter, nanny/au pair, parent in another home, grandparents, and eventually school, our children will be influenced elsewhere.

Providing a solid foundation at home and knowing how to get others "on board" will be an invaluable asset. This section will provide some help with how to get your other "educators" on board with your nutrition goals.

We haven't overlooked your most invaluable asset – your kids! We've listed a couple of pointers on dealing with the inevitable peer pressure that affects their food choices, how to grocery shop with your children (can you say, "NO"), and how to make gathering groceries a little more fun.

## Parental Modeling

The short and sweet of it is that you are the best role model for your children! If you have a healthy attitude toward food and exercise, chances are your children will too. Raise their nutrition and fitness IQ while you can (at least when they slack off in college, they'll have a healthy foundation to fall back on).

The more informed and confident they are about why they eat certain foods and not others, the more likely they will be to make good choices when they are away from you.

If you have issues about food, try to resolve them before you pass them on to your children. Don't be afraid of letting them know you've made mistakes, but be willing to step up to the plate when they ask, "Mommy, why do you get to eat three donuts and I don't?"

## Blended Family Life

Many of our children are living with two parents in two separate households. Make sure you have a conversation with the "ex" about the fact that you want your kids' diet to be as consistent as possible while they are living at each home. This may be stretching it, but it is worth trying.

Consider some of the following points brought up by a friend who has experience with blended family life:

- Make sure to establish common goals about their health, education, religion, etc. – if you can. Try to discuss your children's doctor appointments, dentist appointments, and progress in school. Discuss the importance of maintaining the same habits and schedule at both homes.

- You might even think about having a Nutrition Tracking Board in each home so your kids can stay on the same track wherever they are. The key to honesty and fairness when it comes to what your kids are eating is simple – communication, which might not be so easy.

- Get on the same page about television, activities, and making sure the children have some form of exercise every day. Talk about what you are cooking and what you eat, and try to have the same kinds of foods in the pantry at each house.

- If all of this is a lot of wishful thinking, then just try to steer clear and do the best you can when they are under your roof!

Be supportive of your children's body image and talk with them
about the importance of "being kind to their bodies."
If you are healthy, then you are the right size!

## Involving Grandparents

Let's face it, our grandparents' generation ate remarkably different from both our parents and us. We need to recognize the culture that each group came from in order to understand where their ideas about nutrition originated.

If I had to leave my kids with my grandmother, they'd be likely to get homemade gelatin salad and some sliced tomatoes for lunch, while my mother is more likely to serve them processed food and wildly colored ketchup. My mother remembers clearly when the first processed food came out and how exciting it was!

If your mother (your child's grandparent) is in the baby boomer generation, then they might not view food and nutrition in the same manner you do. If you are reading this book, it's likely you and your own grandmother would have a more similar approach to food and nutrition.

Just be gentle. You might not want to take my route and end up in a screaming match with your father-in-law about why you are wasting good money on organic milk, or the other fun time when my mother fed my toddlers an entire array of chocolate and pop tarts for breakfast. (I left the house and allowed her to deal with the inevitable meltdowns.)

Try to understand their side, and try to be reasonable in overcoming whatever food nonsense that generation got fed with. They were sold on nutrients as something far removed from whole food, as well as the idea that you could use convenience foods to improve your life!

If you have grandparents, parents, or in-laws that share your goals about healthy eating, then they will be an invaluable asset. Many grandparents have gotten Nutrition Tracking Boards for their grandchildren.

For those that don't necessarily share your goals about what is good for the kids to eat, we have a couple of suggestions:

- Let it be known that you are working to teach your children how to eat healthy and why, and that you want to raise healthy grandchildren for them.

- Make sure you both understand that a little treat here and there is OK, but they don't need to win your children's hearts by going through their stomachs.

- You can always offer to help fix heathier foods. Provide some healthy snacks rather than mandating what they should fix.

- Try not to put down anyone's dietary habits – it only gets the issue off track. You can really only control what you are doing anyway, and your children's grandparents certainly aren't "yours to raise." There's a bad country song and a healthy life lesson in there somewhere.

- As with everything, keep the big picture in mind.

## Involving Caregivers

When your kids are in the care of others on a regular basis, try to explain the importance of the healthy choices you are making. One of the most important things you will teach your children is how to take care of their bodies. Their caregivers should share your philosophy as much as possible. Recruit them as an ally in teaching healthy habits.

Give them good information, if they don't have it. And if they are responsible for grocery shopping for your family, make certain they are willing to "shop healthy."

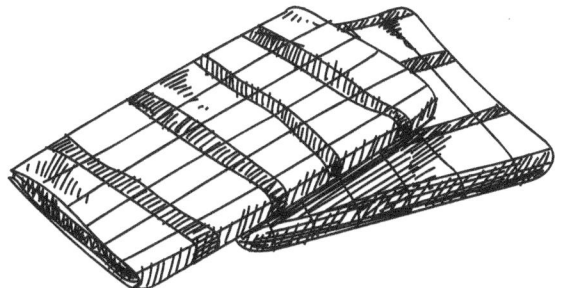

# School Lunch

If your kids are of school age, they are getting at least a third of their daily intake away from you. You are either packing a lunch for them to take or hoping they will be eating healthy choices from the school cafeteria. In either case, you want to give them good information that they can use to make good decisions about their choices when they are not at home.

## Eating the School Lunch

If your child eats lunches provided by the school, figure out what they are actually offering and if it is suitable. Most schools have contracts with a major food supplier that will have stringent guidelines about the food they are serving. This doesn't always mean that it is going to be the best option available.

If your school publishes their menus in advance, be sure to talk with your children about what they would like to eat (if they have the option of packing their lunches some days) in order to give them some decision-making power. Use your Nutrition Tracking Board to discuss why they need to eat their veggies and drink their milk each time they sit down for lunch. Keep in mind that school menus might change from the printed versions that are sent out.

Try to have lunch with your child one day to see what their experience is like. If you feel like you need to encourage healthier choices, try to talk to your school's lunch provider personally. Ask the school administration how you can engage lunch providers in a dialogue about what they are serving.

Always have the attitude that you want to help and partner with them to make sure the kids are getting fresh foods and limits on sweets.

## The Lunch Box Gang

If you are sending your kids to school with a lunch box, try to keep these things in mind.

- Let them be involved in packing their lunches – they will be more likely to eat what they have chosen.

- Try to do it the night before if you can so you aren't making decisions on the fly in the morning with only one eye open.

**Keep lunches cold if you include any perishable foods, especially mayonnaise!**

If you are depending on "lunchable" type meals – ready to serve and waiting patiently in your grocer's fridge – then please read the back of the packaging to see what you are actually serving your kids, nutritionally speaking. Golly, didn't realize I'd gotten up on that soapbox again!

If your kids only want to eat the same thing each day, more power to them – as long as it is balanced and healthy! If you would like some inspiration about how to pack a healthier variety, there are hundreds of blogs and other fantastic resources online. (Let your kids check them out with you.)

Try to offer foods that are easy to eat quickly (as our nutritionist Emily Harrison mentioned in the Fruit portion of the Nutrition section). Peel and section oranges, and cut fruit and veggies into bite-sized pieces or "sticks."

Knowing what your kids are actually eating at school isn't always easy. You could pack the best, most nutritious lunch on the planet, and they might not eat it all, might toss half of it, might trade with a friend, etc. Try to encourage them to bring home what they don't eat so you can tell what they are consuming. Make sure you aren't judgmental about it after the fact, or they will end up "dumping it" rather than face the wrath of the finger-shakin' parent.

## Peer Pressure

It is out there in a huge way. Not only for our children but for us too – checked social media lately? If you are able to equip your kids with the knowledge they need about nutrition and why a balanced diet makes your body look and feel better, then they will be better equipped to deal with peer pressure and the food issues that result. A strong foundation will go miles towards improving their success – let them know it is cool to eat well!

School-age kids will eventually become body conscious, and it will affect their eating habits. Practice our mantra: If you are healthy, then you will be the "right size."

If you are concerned that your child may be getting too self-conscious or developing other eating issues, speak to your family doctor, get some help from a registered dietitian, and check out this website: www.myedin.org. The Eating Disorders Information Network has some great information about dealing with this issue, including suggestions for how dads can support their daughters to develop healthy eating habits! (How many of us are still dragging around an off-hand comment a parent made when we were pre-teen, suggesting that we "might be getting a little chubby"?)

Pay attention to foods that might be "socially uncomfortable" for kids to take to school. Lunch classics like tuna fish or egg salad (along with being served with mayonnaise, which needs to stay cold for safety reasons) also have a very strong odor. If your child tells you they don't like to have those foods because the other kids call them "stinky," then listen to them. There is plenty of time on weekends or evenings for them to eat those very nutritious foods. You can pack the best egg salad sandwich on the planet, but if your child is socially uncomfortable about eating it, it will stay in their lunchbox or go directly into the trash can.

We should encourage our children not to bow down to peer pressure, but the bottom line is that they will encounter it at some point. We all pay attention to how we look. How we look is very much related to what we eat and how much exercise we get. If you are able to equip your kids with the knowledge they need about nutrition, and why a good balanced diet makes your body look and feel better, then they will be better equipped to deal with peer pressure and health issues later in life. A strong foundation will go miles toward improving their success – let them know it is cool to eat well!

# Choosing Your Meals

*How To Say NO in the Grocery Store*

How about, "NO!" If you don't know this already, we'll let you in on a well-kept secret that you only find out postpartum: you are actually required to say "NO" about 300 times a day. Another well-kept secret that is imparted only after you've committed parenthood: grocery shopping with your children will make you cry. You will also bring home six bags of cookies you'd never, in your younger (more stable) mind, have given the time of day.

Your biggest ally in the grocery store will be an educated child. Give them knowledge about why foods are healthy and a list of "good choices" they get to make, and have them search for their "good choices" in the store. If they are too young to read, you can tell them what items they need to find. "Can you pick out our bananas today?" Or, "Could you choose a bottle of juice from THIS shelf?" (Pick a shelf with the healthiest, lowest sugar choices.)

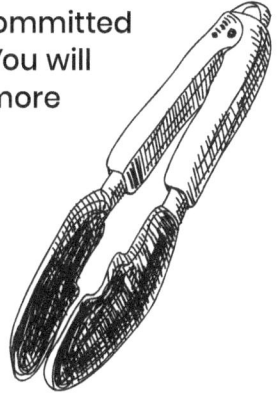

Give them a chance to make choices – just pick what they get to choose from. In the cereal aisle for instance, let them know which three cereals they can choose from. If they start to get really whiny about another kind and don't want to choose from the selection you gave them, then you will choose for them. (Or put said whine-inducing items in the cart and secretly slip it to the cashier with a silent "sorry," and hope you can finish the checkout before your child realizes it ain't coming home. Kidding! ...Maybe.)

When they are old enough, let them read the labels. When they realize that there are 41g of sugar in one brand of "low-fat" yogurt and 12 in another – or they stumble over pronouncing the list of ingredients because each word is actually a chemical compound – they will begin to understand what you are talking about.

Don't be afraid to have other people hear you establish control. Other adults in the grocery store will not point fingers at you. They've either been there themselves or they have worse habits than you do. Remaining silent to try and keep a polite face on things does not create a teaching moment. The goal is always to get your shopping done without having a major crying fit (you or your children).

Make sure they understand that if it gets to be too unpleasant to continue shopping, then you will have to leave the store. Then you will have no groceries! I've even said, "We will have to go tell the store manager that we have to leave, and hope they don't get upset about the full grocery cart they will have to re-shelve." (I know, I know – the guilt thing!) Hopefully, when they understand that their behavior will make you have to leave with no groceries, they will choose to continue shopping in a civilized manner. If not, then you have to leave. Insert crying fit here... Under no circumstances should you go through the drive-thru to get dinner that night. Find something scary to serve from the back of the pantry!

## Where to Shop – Make Shopping for Food Fun

Food doesn't come from a grocery store! Yes, I know that sounds ridiculous, because it absolutely does come from a grocery store, and we love our Publix, but REAL food at its most nutritious comes from a farm. Teach your children the value of fresh foods by introducing them to a local farm or farmers market. They will love it, and you will be giving them a valuable lesson about where foods really come from.

Join a CSA! With a Community Supported Agriculture program, you will be supporting your local farms so they can grow fresh foods close to your home. Remember: the closer you eat food to its natural state (not processed or shipped from across the globe), the better the foods are for your body, and the smaller the environmental impact will be. Ask them if you can visit the farm one day.

Check out this phenomenal national resource: www.localharvest.org. Just plug in your ZIP code, and it will give you a listing of local organic farms, farmers markets, organic restaurants, and more great resources!

This section is short but it is tremendously important! Find, buy, and eat REAL FOOD. A great tidbit I gleaned from Michael Pollan's book, *In Defense of Food*, is to only buy what your grandmother or great-grandmother would have recognized as food. That means twinkies and purple ketchup are out.

## Dining Out?

Try to choose restaurants that offer healthy choices for your children. Typical kid menus include hamburgers, chicken fingers, and french fries. Choose restaurants that put a vegetable on the plate rather than automatically plopping down a load of french fries. Restaurants most likely put fries on the plate because they are inexpensive and easy. Serving a fresh veg might be more difficult, but the payoff could be very valuable for a restaurant in the long run. Let them know you might pay a bit more for good choices. Reward their good behavior by visiting often. And remember, mac and cheese is not a veg!

We frequent a local noodle house because they have great choices for the kids. Broccoli and carrots are part of their kids' dishes – it isn't just an option! We appreciate it, Doc Chey's (www.doccheys.com).

If you know of a restaurant that you would recommend based on these ideas, let us know! We'd love to shout about them on social media.

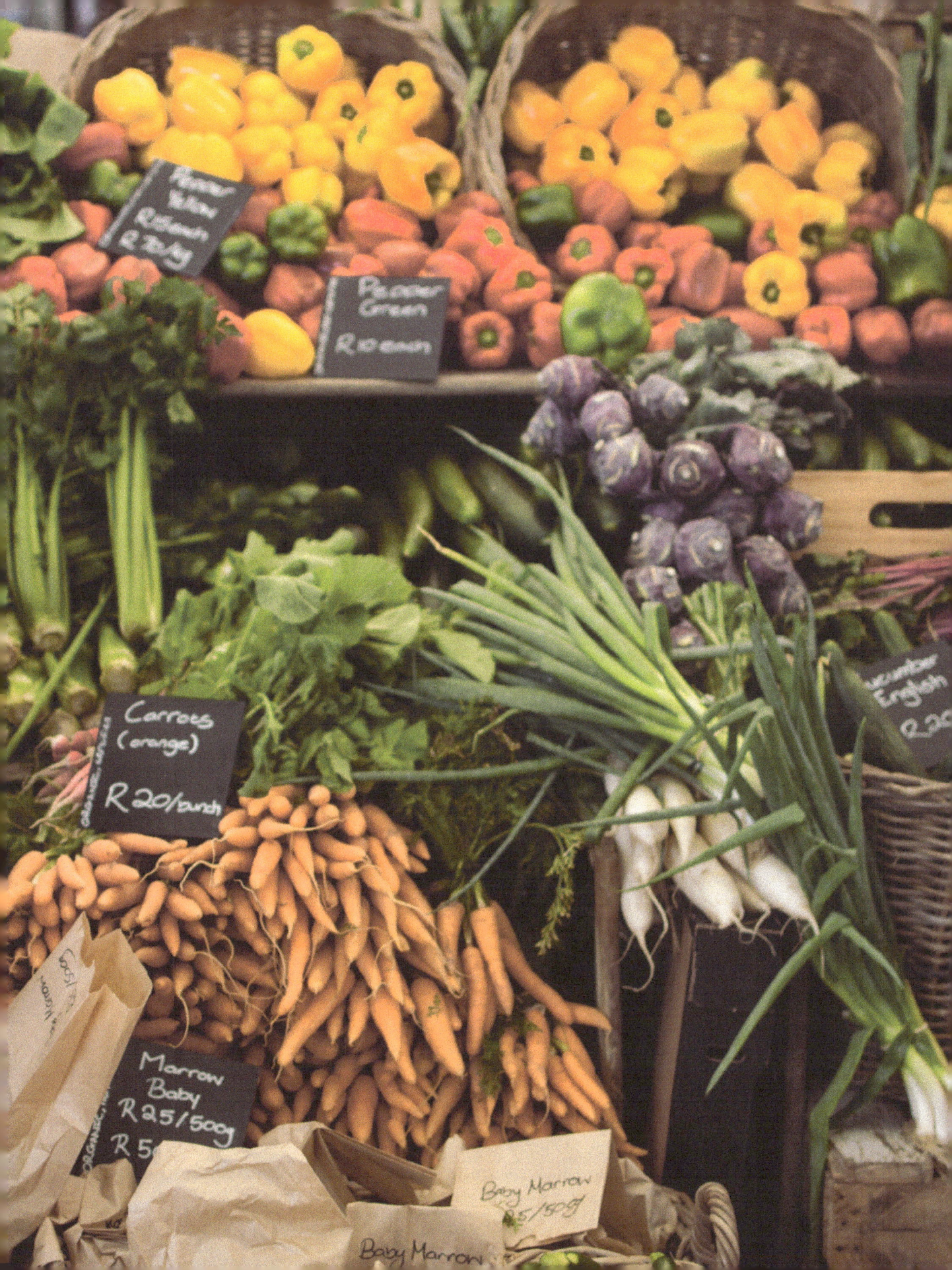

Pepper Yellow
Ribbish
R 25/kg

Pepper
Green
R 10 each

Carrots
(orange)

R 20/bunch

cucumber
English
R 20

Marrow
Baby
R 25/500g

R 5

Baby Marrow
R25/500g

Baby Marrow

# About Us

Lending expertise are several talented friends/neighbors/parents who have joined in the mission to help busy modern families teach their own kids about good nutrition and staying active.

## Leslie Smith Grant

Leslie Grant currently serves on the Atlanta Board of Education and works a part-time gig in the Center for Mind, Brain, and Culture at Emory University. From 2007-2012, she was the "Mother Hen" of Chickin Feed, LLC, a small business she created to help her family focus on raising healthy kids (chickins) from scratch. She wanted a simple, fun way for her kids to make wise decisions about what they were eating, as well as something to help her figure out what to make for dinner each night. Leslie and her "chicken coop" of talented friends released the original edition of this book in 2008, The Chickin Feed Primer, after appearing as the first "Incredible People" on the Rachael Ray Show. Chickin Feed, LLC also produced a series of books and a collection of children's tunes based upon a quirky set of Farm Grub characters. If you email her, she might just let you know how to find some Chickin Feed. (LeslieSmithGrant@gmail.com)

Leslie was involved in the startup of both the Neighborhood Charter School in Grant Park (now the K-8, Atlanta Neighborhood Charter School) and the Grant Park Cooperative Preschool, and has served on the boards of each school. She has volunteered in Farm to School programs through work with Georgia Organics, Atlanta Farm to School, the Grant Park Farmers Market, and other organizations. As a member of the Atlanta Board of Education, she serves as the chairperson of the Audit Committee and on the Executive Committee of the Council of Great City Schools. Leslie is very impressed by her ability to stay married to Don and the two great chickins they've raised.

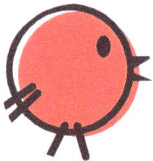

## Emily Harrison / Nutrition

Emily keeps nutrition and health a priority in all that we do. Emily is a registered dietitian and holds both a bachelor's and master's degree in nutrition from Georgia State University. She was formerly a principal ballet dancer with the Atlanta Ballet as well as on the faculty with the Atlanta Ballet Centre for Dance Education. She ran the Centre for Dance Nutrition and Healthy Lifestyles at Atlanta Ballet for 6 years.

Emily has also worked in the clinical nutrition department of Children's Healthcare of Atlanta: Scottish Rite as a nutrition technician and at Peachford Behavioral Health Center in the eating disorder unit and the child and adolescent unit. She is a member of the American Dietetic Association and the Greater Atlanta Dietetic Association. Emily teaches ballet to the neighborhood kids. She is a mother of two who uses this book with her own kids and understands the unique challenges parents face when it comes to feeding children, especially ones with food allergies. Emily runs a private practice, Dancer Nutrition (DancerNutrition.com), where she provides nutrition counseling for atheletes and families, and also works on various community nutrition projects in Atlanta.

## Sheri Davis / Chef

Sheri develops tasty, kid-friendly recipes and menus. She had a long and devout following in Atlanta as co-owner and executive chef of the former Virginia-Highland restaurant Dish, which emphasized fresh, seasonal, and locally grown products. Sheri is the chef-owner of a very successful catering business called Fresh World Cuisine with her husband Vando.

Before opening Dish, Sheri was the opening sous chef at Atlanta's much-loved Harvest restaurant. She came to Atlanta via Milwaukee, Wisconsin where she started her cooking career at the James Beard Award-winning restaurant, Sanford. From there Sheri traveled to San Francisco and New York, working at the Quilted Giraffe and the famed Le Bernardin, and she finally made her way south to open Brassiere Le Coze in Atlanta in 1994. She is the mother of two fine young men.

## Randy Brookins / P.E. Coach

Randy creates exciting activities to keep kids moving. Formerly at Atlanta Neighborhood Charter School, where he was known as Coach Brookins, Randy graduated with a master's degree in Health and Physical Education from the University of Georgia. While at ANCS, he taught elementary physical education and language arts, was recognized with both the school and district Teacher of the Year Award in 1999, and was a nominee for the Teacher of the Year for the State of Georgia. He currently teaches at The Children's School. He is actively involved in community youth sports and cultural arts programs, and he can often be overheard encouraging his students (and their parents) to stay active.

## Amy Handler / Drama

Amy designs fun, dramatic ways for kids to stay active. Amy earned a BA degree in performing arts and art history at Washington University in St. Louis, and an MFA in Children's Theatre at the University of Texas at Austin. Even in college she pursued her two loves – teaching drama and children's television. She spent two summers working at Nick Jr., where she worked on the pilot for and helped develop Blue's Clues. She also developed cartoons for Cartoon Network for six years. Her experience as a drama teacher spans from pre-K to college, but her greatest love is using drama as a tool to teach other subjects. She can be found entertaining the masses in archives of The Kids are Alright radio series (exchange.prx.org).

## Michelle Newcome / Editor

Michelle makes sense out of chaos on a daily basis, and she has the privilege of making a living telling other people what to do as an expert in crisis management and organizational resilience. She is the CEO of White Deer Group and publisher of How2Conquer. Michelle has somewhat successfully parented two children out of her roost and into adulthood.

# Links and Resources

This resource list includes things we liked and found helpful. We do not suggest endorsement of Rule a Healthy Roost by any of these folks – we just think they are grand for some reason or another. There are plenty more resources available. Search the web to find some that work for your family. Print out helpful information and keep it in a notebook that you make with your kids .

Remember: Don't spend more time looking for information to use than you do actually enjoying the fruits of your research!

## *Recipe websites & cookbooks*

- **www.epicurious.com** – The Bon Appétit and Gourmet Magazine folks.

- **www.foodnetwork.com** – Check out their kid-friendly products.

- **www.americastestkitchen.com** – You will get a rich lesson in the art of cooking and make some incredible recipes. From the PBS show America's Test Kitchen.

- **www.missvickie.com** – Fabulous compendium of everything pressure-cooker.

- *Culinary Artistry* by Andrew Dornenburg and Karen Page. Extensive lists of which foods marry well and which are mortal enemies. Great book for aspiring chefs and foodies.

- *Greene on Greens* by Bert Greene. Everything you ever wanted to know about vegetables and how to cook them.

- *The Grains Cookbook* by Bert Greene. Want to get more whole foods and good grains into your diet? This exhaustive book covers every major grain, including history and how to cook. Each grain has a recipe section.

- *In Defense of Food: An Eater's Manifesto* by Michael Pollan. Check out his other titles on www.amazon.com.

- *Slow Food Nation: Why Our Food Should Be Good, Clean, and Fair* by Carlo Petrini with foreward by Alice Waters.

- *Atlanta Cooks at Home* by Melissa Libby, photography by Joey Ivansco and Tim Wilkerson. Our very own Chef Chick, Sheri Davis, is featured in this book.

- ***Sugar Busters! Quick & Easy Cookbook*** by H. Leighton Steward, Morrison Bethea MD, Sam Andrews MD, and Luis Balart MD.

- ***How to Eat: The Pleasures and Principles of Good Food*** by Nigella Lawson. Great section on how to feed children, with some very kid-friendly and healthy options.

- ***Rachael Ray Yum-O: The Family Cookbook*** by Rachael Ray. Her Yum-O foundation empowers kids and their families to develop healthy relationships with food and cooking.

## Nutrition & Fitness Resources

- **www.eatright.org** – Visit the Food tab for good resources from the heart of the Academy of Nutrition and Dietetics. You can also search the site to find a registered dietitian.

- **www.nps.gov** – Home of the National Park Service. Look up your state park service or local department of parks and recreation to find a park close by. Find a great place, pack healthy snacks, put something in the crock pot and go! Find out if there is a park conservancy program in your area and volunteer with your chickens!

## More Cool Stuff

- **bentology.com** – A fantastic resource for helping plan and pack nutritious school lunches and a way to keep millions of pounds of lunch waste out of landfills. Our favorite part is the photos of healthy lunches – lots of variety!

- **www.edibleschoolyard.org** – Want to get really inspired? Check out this website from Alice Waters, the mother of the organic/slow foods movement.

- **www.flylady.com** – The ultimate resource for organizing your life and giving you back enough time to actually cook a decent meal.

- **www.foodsafety.gov** – Lots of information about food contamination, foodborne illness and how to cook safely.

# Acknowledgements

I would like to gratefully acknowledge all who contributed – in large part or small – to this book.

I would like to thank my husband Don for being my most important person. His help and support in this enterprise has been critical. Thank you from the bottom of my heart – I love you. Thank you so much to my beloved chickens, Lucy and Will, for your pride in and patience with your mom and her "chicken business." Thanks to Pop Pop Troy, Miles, and Keith for bankrolling this crazy idea. Thanks to Deb Elkin for showing me that I had the power to go home all along.

Thank you to Michelle Newcome, who created order out of chaos and didn't laugh at all when I told her we needed to write a book. Thank you to Sonia Fuller for using her amazing PR powers for good. Thank you to Emily Harrison for immediately "getting it." Thank you to Coach Brookins for keeping our chickens active. Thank you to Amy Handler for bringing the fun. Thank you to Chef Sheri Davis for enthusiastically coming in to play late in the fourth quarter! Thanks to the chickens: Isabelle, Telia and Joel, Jake and Luke and baby Riles, Eleanor, Manhattan ( chicken-dog), Oliver and Calliope, Vando and Dione, and Lydia and Quincy for sharing your families.

Thank you to Tomas Clements for being the "host with the most." Thank you to Matthew Drooker for always coming through with hardware and parking spots! Thank you to Stephanie Ricker and Leslie Hudson for your enthusiastic participation. Thank you to Clay Pullen for saying, "Sure, we can do that," when I asked him to make the boards. Thank you to Melanie Manning at Belly General Store who said, "Sure, we can sell those," when I showed her the boards.

Thanks to Ann Brewster and Kim Evatt for being great friends and buying the first boards. (I know you had to, but thanks anyway!) Thank you to the parents in our great community of Grant Park who provide insight and support each day. Thanks to our chicken Testers (Michael Berzsenyi, Lynn Brandli, and Stacy Phillips).

Thanks to all of the inspirational women entrepreneurs and all the other fabulous folks we've met along the way who are following their passion or enjoying ours!

Cheers,
Leslie Smith Grant

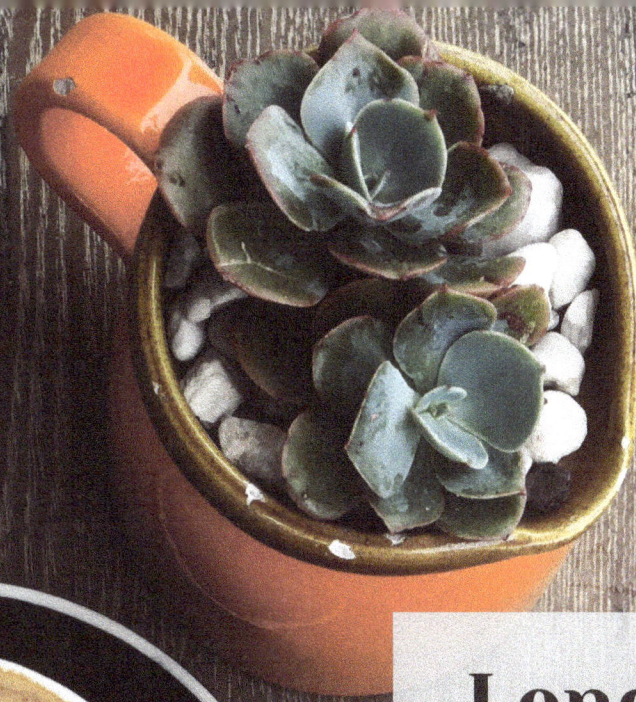

Lend this
book to a
friend!

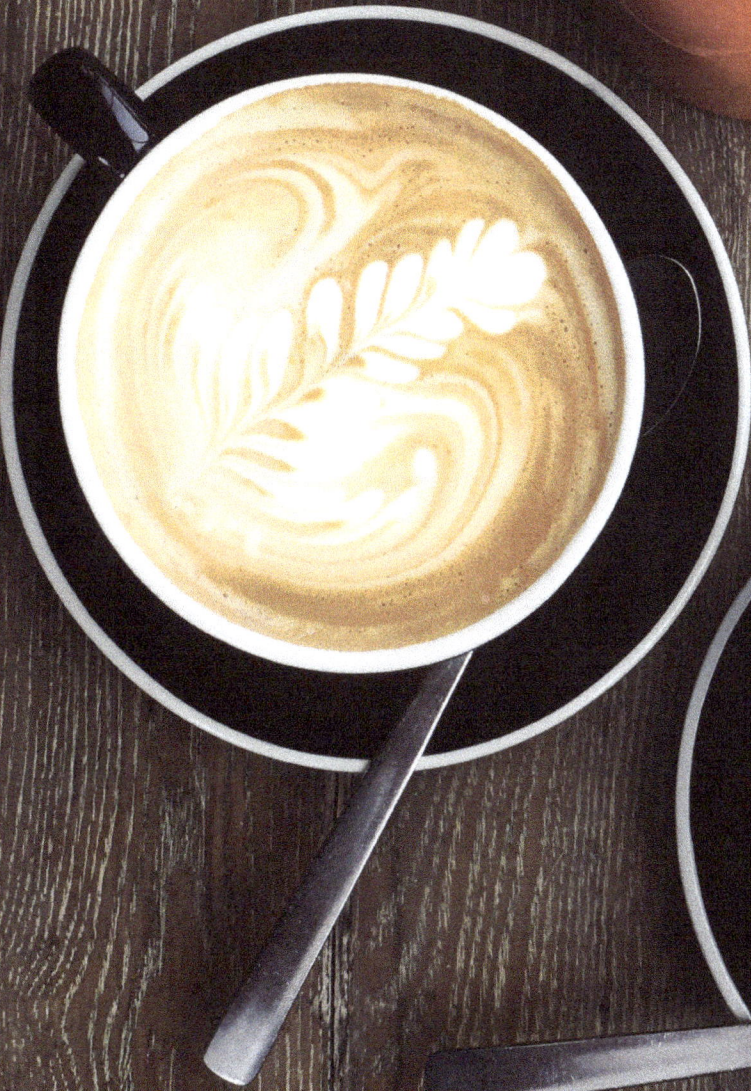

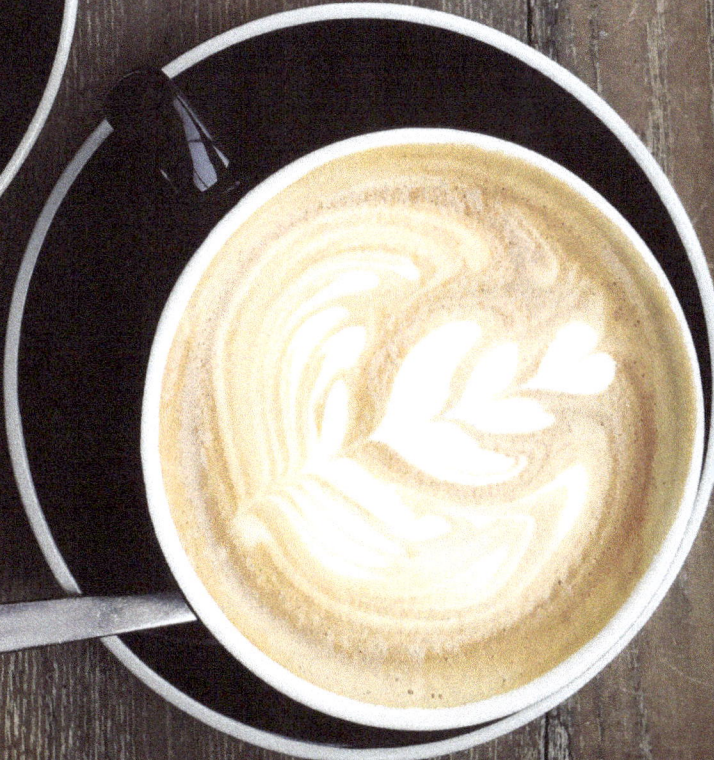

www.ingramcontent.com/pod-product-compliance
Lightning Source LLC
Chambersburg PA
CBHW051315020426
42333CB00028B/3350